Trauma Practice

About the Authors

Anna B. Baranowsky, PhD, CPsych is a registered clinical psychologist and the Founder and director of Traumatology Institute (Canada). She was instrumental in co-developing training materials for the Traumatology Institute Training Curriculum (TITC). She is the developer of ww.ticlearn.com, the online training site for the TITC. Dr. Baranowsky received her doctorate in Clinical Psychology at the University of Ottawa. Her accomplishments include the co-development of the Accelerated Recovery Program (ARP) for Compassion Fatigue, National and International presentations on the ARP, trauma assessment, treatment, and interventions. She has published in the area of secondary traumatization, compassion fatigue, the ARP and therapeutic relationships (the Silencing Response). Dr. Baranowsky serves on the Board of Directors of the Academy of Traumatology's Commission on Certification and Accreditation. She has been recognized by the American Academy of Experts in Traumatic Stress with Diplomate status and is a Board Certified Expert in Traumatic Stress. Dr. Baranowsky dedicates a large portion of her clinical practice to care for the emotional well-being of trauma survivors. She has been trained in many cutting-edge trauma treatments now being recognized as highly effective in resolving the emotional aftermath of exposure to trauma. Dr. Baranowsky works with a wide range of trauma survivors from airplane crash survivors to victims of violence as well as first responders at trauma scenes. Her dedication to the emotional recovery of survivors is witnessed in her passion for training others to gain skills to work effectively in the newly emerging field of Traumatology.
info@psychink.com

J. Eric Gentry, PhD, LMHC is an internationally recognized leader in the study and treatment of traumatic stress and compassion fatigue. His doctorate is from Florida State University where he studied with Professor Charles Figley, a pioneer in the fields of traumatic stress and compassion fatigue. Gentry has worked with hundreds of professional caregivers from all over the world to help them recover from work-related symptoms. He has also worked with many of the volunteers and professionals affected following their work with disaster survivors, including the Oklahoma, New York, and many natural disasters. He is in his 28th year as a professional caregiver/clinician and maintains a private psychotherapy practice in Sarasota. He has trained tens of thousands of international caregiving professionals through Compassion Unlimited, his private training/consulting practice, and through his tenure as Associate Director of the original Traumatology Institute at FSU and as Co-Director of the International Traumatology Institute at the University of South Florida. He has published many research articles, book chapters, and periodicals on the topics of traumatic stress and compassion fatigue treatment/resiliency.
eg@compassionunlimited.com

D. Franklin Schultz, PhD is a clinical psychologist in private practice in Lakeland, Florida. He is an adjunct faculty member at Webster University, where he teaches graduate classes in personality and psychotherapy. Dr. Schultz is also the author of *A Language of the Heart: Therapy Stories That Heal* (www.ALOTH.com) and *A Language of the Heart Workbook*. He provides workshops and trainings on stress management and communications in corporate, military, and private settings. He is a Master Traumatologist, certified compassion fatigue specialist, a member of Green Cross, and past clinical director and board president of the Polk County (Florida) Critical Incident Stress Management Team.
drfrank@aloth.com

Trauma Practice
Tools for Stabilization and Recovery

2nd revised and expanded edition

Anna B. Baranowsky, PhD, CPsych
J. Eric Gentry, PhD, LMHC
D. Franklin Schultz, PhD

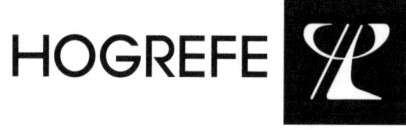

Library of Congress Cataloging-in-Publication Data
is available via the Library of Congress Marc Database under the
LC Control Number 2010933543

Library and Archives Canada Cataloguing in Publication
Baranowsky, Anna B., 1961-
 Trauma practice : tools for stabilization and recovery / Anna B. Baranowsky, J. Eric Gentry, D. Franklin Schultz. -- 2nd rev. and expanded ed.

Includes bibliographical references.
ISBN 978-0-88937-380-8

 1. Post-traumatic stress disorder--Treatment. 2. Psychic trauma--Treatment. I. Schultz, D. Franklin, 1952- II. Gentry, J. Eric III. Title.

RC552.P67B37 2010   616.85'2106   C2010-905416-4

© 2011 by Hogrefe Publishing

PUBLISHING OFFICES
USA: Hogrefe Publishing, 875 Massachusetts Avenue, 7th Floor, Cambridge, MA 02139
 Phone (866) 823-4726, Fax (617) 354-6875, E-mail customerservice@hogrefe-publishing.com
EUROPE: Hogrefe Publishing, Rohnsweg 25, 37085 Göttingen, Germany
 Phone +49 551 49609-0, Fax +49 551 49609-88, E-mail publishing@hogrefe.com

SALES & DISTRIBUTION
USA: Hogrefe Publishing, Customer Services Department, 30 Amberwood Parkway, Ashland, OH 44805
 Phone (800) 228-3749, Fax (419) 281-6883, E-mail customerservice@hogrefe.com
EUROPE: Hogrefe Publishing, Rohnsweg 25, 37085 Göttingen, Germany
 Phone +49 551 49609-0, Fax +49 551 49609-88, E-mail publishing@hogrefe.com

OTHER OFFICES
CANADA: Hogrefe Publishing, 660 Eglinton Ave. East, Suite 119-514, Toronto, Ontario, M4G 2K2
SWITZERLAND: Hogrefe Publishing, Länggass-Strasse 76, CH-3000 Bern 9

Hogrefe Publishing
Incorporated and registered in the Commonwealth of Massachusetts, USA, and in Göttingen, Lower Saxony, Germany

No part of this book may be reproduced, stored in a retrieval system or transmitted, in any form or by any means, electronic, mechanical, photocopying, microfilming, recording or otherwise, without written permission from the publisher.

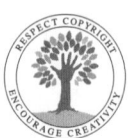

Printed and bound in the USA
ISBN 978-0-88937-380-8

Foreword

This book, *Trauma Practice: Tools for Stabilization and Recovery*, represents a new generation of resources for traumatologists – those who study or treat the traumatized. A good indication of this comes in the first few chapters of background and history, because by now the assessment and treatment of the traumatized are far from novel.

Today we know that traumatic stress desensitization treatments work. We know that exposure to the conditioned (fear) stimulus is a critical element to the treatment, the primary active ingredient. We also know that clients' ability to tolerate exposure to what they fear varies greatly and that it is counterproductive, if not a breach of professional standards of practice, to not offer the most gentle ways for clients to reach the therapeutic threshold for such exposure.

We know today that iatrogenic effects of trauma therapy are real and that practitioners must be extraordinarily cautious when interviewing the client, developing a treatment plan, and insuring that there is sufficient safety as well as retraumatization containment strategies. Remission is expected and, therefore, relapse prevention training is a requirement.

We also know that the assessment of the traumatized is not an exact science. Extraordinary events that would traumatize most people have little effect on some. Conversely, exposure to rather noxious stimuli can cause extraordinary traumatic stress reactions for others. Children tend to be rather hardy and spring back with apparently no negative effects. Their parents, on the other hand, have lingering symptoms. Although women appear more symptomatic, war-related PTSD is actually less frequent in them than in men.

Clients with PTSD are very challenging. Most PTSD clients, for example, are dual diagnosed. It is rare to find clients with PTSD who do *not* have at least one additional diagnosis. Often, it is another anxiety disorder or depression. Often, both are seen in addition to PTSD. Very often when a client is diagnosed with a drug dependency, she or he is also diagnosed with PTSD.

All this we know, and this important book both addresses what we know today at a theoretical level and, equally importantly, explains clinical methods in the context of treatment. More than the typical book about why and how the cognitive behavioral treatment approaches work, Baranowsky, Gentry, & Schultz offer a comprehensive guide for clinicians working with the traumatized. This book presents clear instructions to traumatologists – even the most experienced in working with the traumatized – to help the traumatized. The guidance is detailed. The authors direct practitioners to focus on symptoms of the body as well as on behavior and emotions associated with trauma. They also link their guidance to a triphasic treatment model that starts with establishing Safety, continues through enabling Trauma Memory Processing, and ends with Reconnection. This book is also an excellent resource for trainers, teachers, and educators of trauma practitioners, providing a how-to manual to address the challenges of clinical traumatology.

These authors represent the current and future generation of clinical traumatologists who are well-equipped to handle the extraordinary challenges of traumatized clients. We have come a long way in ten years, as illustrated by this useful book.

Charles R. Figley, PhD
Florida State University Traumatology Institute
Tallahassee, July 2010

Acknowledgments

Anna B. Baranowsky – To my beloved parents who taught me love and life exists even after terrible losses. To my dear husband Chris, my compassionate warrior and companion in all life's joys and of course, to Cassi, our cherished Chow-Lab, who joined us in adventures for 13 happy years. To Dr. Michael McCarrey, the greatest of mentors and friends. To Marlene Mawhinney and B.K.S Iyengar, my yoga teachers of over 20 years, whose work has brought me the harmony and resiliency which allows me to do this remarkable work. Big thanks to Gold for playtime and being an extended family. To my wonderful inspiring writer's group, Doug, Monica, and Joanne; to Evan and the Mastermind group for ongoing focus. To Maureen and Judit, who help me with everything and do so with enormous grace – I am forever appreciative of your efforts. To my practice colleagues at Sheppard Yonge Psychological Services, who make it a good place to be. I am grateful to Dr. Charles Figley for laying fertile ground at just the perfect time. Special thanks to D. Franklin Schultz for his essential contributions to this manuscript. To my friend and inspiration, Eric, who willingly joins me in challenging dialogue and laughter. Mostly, to my clients, students, trainers, and friends over the years who have taught me more than they could imagine and helped me stay humble and continue to learn and grow ... I am grateful.

J. Eric Gentry – Thanks go to the mentors in my life in order of their appearance: Charles "Charlie" Yeargan, PhD; Louis Tinnin, MD; Charles Figley, PhD; and Michael Rank, PhD. Gratitude to N. A. and H. P. for keeping me alive long enough to write this work. Thanks to my support, in no particular order: Marjie, Diane, Mom, Bubbita, Augie, MaryJoan, PDR, Mason, Rosalina, TZap, Jennifer, Dane, Connor, Frank, Jim "Big Bro" Norman, Carlos & Family, Eduardo & Maria, Jim Hussey, Joe Williams, Nacho & Lucy, ITI Site Directors, Melissa, and my family. A special mention of gratitude for the creative and supportive relationship that I share with Anna – you are the BEST! I dedicate this text to all my clients and trainees – past, present, and future.

D. Franklin Schultz – As is usual in any undertaking such as this, there are many more who contribute to the final outcome than the ones who have their names on it. First and foremost I would like to thank my clients, who have taught me every bit as much as I them. There is an incredible amount of healing that occurs in the therapist in the course of any work with another. For that healing and learning I am very grateful. And, I have been graced with a wonderful series of mentors in my life. These are individuals who stand out for their dedication to their ideals, their desire to see those around them grow, and the love with which they foster it. These are: my dad, David Schultz, Dr. Donn Baumann, Dr. Kathleen Adams, Dr. Sydnor Sikes, Dr. Jev Sikes, and Dr. Eric Gentry. Each of them provided a crucial piece of understanding to my development as a therapist. I also would like to thank my mentor, my friend, my wife and lover, Lori, for accompanying me in this adventure. And finally, thanks to both Dr. Anna Baranowsky and, again, Dr. Eric Gentry for asking me to participate in this endeavor. Working with them is delightful.

Dedication

This text is dedicated to unsung heroes, the caregivers who maintain the courage and the stamina to bear witness to the stories and selves of trauma survivors, making healing a reality.

See first that you yourself deserve to be a giver,
and an instrument of giving.
For in truth it is life that gives unto life –
while you, who deem yourself a giver,
are but a witness.
Khalil Gibran

Table of Contents

Foreword v
Acknowledgments vi

Introduction: Trauma Practice: Tools for Stabilization and Recovery 1
    Purpose of This Book 3
    Self-of-the-Therapist 4
    Core Objectives 4
    Book Description 5
    Supportive Texts and Other Recommended Readings 6

Section 1: Foundations of the Trauma Practice Model 7
  1. Behavioral Therapy 10
  2. Cognitive Therapy 14
  3. Cognitive-Behavioral Therapy 15
  4. Cognitive-Behavioral Therapy Research 16
      Expert Guidelines 16
      The International Society for Traumatic Stress Studies (ISTSS) Practice Guidelines .. 16
  5. Psychophysiology of Trauma 18
  6. Tri-Phasic Model 21
      Safety and Stabilization 21
      Trauma Memory Processing 21
      Reconnection 21
  7. Necessary Ingredients – Treatment Codes (R, RE, CR) 22
  8. Body, Cognition, Behavior, and Emotion/Relation 22
  9. Posttrauma Response 23

Section 2: Safety and Stabilization 25
  1. What Is Safety? 28
      Minimum Criterion Required for Transition to Phase II Treatment .. 29
  2. Body 30
      Creating a Nonanxious Presence (R – RE – CR) 30
      Titration Part I: Trigger List Using Braking and Acceleration (R – RE – CR) 34
      Progressive Relaxation (R) 39
      Autogenics (R – CR) 40
      Diaphragmatic Breathing (R) 42
      3-6 Breathing (R) 42
      5-4-3-2-1 Sensory Grounding and Containment (R) 44
      Postural Grounding (R) 44
      Anchoring Part I: Collapsing Anchors (R) 45
  3. Cognition 46
      Anchoring Part II: Safety (R) 46
      Safe-Place Visualization (R) 49
      Positive Self-Talk and Thought Replacement/Transformation (CR) 50
      Flashback Journal (R – RE) 56
      Thought-Stopping (R – RE – CR) 58
      Buddha's Trick (R – CR) 58
  4. Behavior 59
      Rituals (R – CR) 59
      Contract for Safety and Self-Care (R – CR) 62
      Safety Net Plan (R – CR) 64
      Timed and Metered Expression Strategies (R – RE) 66

5. Emotion/Relation 68
   Transitional Objects (R) 68
   Support Systems (R – CR) 68
   Drawing Icon and Envelope (Emotional Containment) (R – RE – CR) 71
   Internal Vault (Emotional Containment) (R – RE – CR) 71
   Positive Hope Box (R – RE – CR) 72

Section 3: Trauma Memory Processing 73
1. Body 76
   Titration Part II: Braking and Acceleration (RE) 76
   Layering (RE – CR) 77
   Comfort in One Part (RE) 80
   A Time-Line Approach (RE – CR) 80
   Biofeedback (R – RE – CR) 81
2. Cognition 82
   Downward Arrow Technique (RE – CR) 82
   Cognitive Continuum (CR) 83
   Calculating True Danger (CR) 86
   Looped Tape Scripting (RE – CR) 87
   Cognitive Processing Therapy (RE – CR) 89
   A Story-Book Approach (RE – CR) 91
   A Written Narrative Approach (RE – CR) 91
3. Behavior 91
   Behavior Change Rehearsal Exercise (RE – CR) 91
   Skills Building Methods (CR) 92
   Imaginal and *In-Vivo* Exposure (RE) 93
   Stress Inoculation Training (RE – CR) 94
   Systematic Desensitization (RE) 99
4. Emotion/Relation 99
   Learning to Be Sad (CR) 100
   Assertiveness Training (CR) 104

Section 4: Reconnection 105
1. Body 108
   Centering (CR) 108
2. Cognition 109
   Exploring Your Cognitive Map (CR) 109
   Victim Mythology (CR) 116
   Letter to Self (CR) 116
3. Behavior 117
   Self-Help and Self-Development (CR) 117
4. Emotion/Relation 117
   Memorials (CR) 118
   Connections with Others (RE – CR) 120

Section 5: Integrative & Clinician Self-Care Models 123
1. The Pinnacle Program: Healing Trauma by Principle-Based Living 126
   Introduction 126
   Phase I: Education 130
   Phase II: Intentionality 140
   Phase III: Practice (Coaching and Desensitization) 146
   Conclusion 148
2. Compassion Fatigue: The Crucible of Transformation 150
   Introduction 150
   Compassion Fatigue: The Crucible of Transformation 150

Compassion Fatigue 151
Accelerated Recovery Program for Compassion Fatigue 154
Compassion Fatigue Specialist Training: Training-as-Treatment 154
Treatment and Prevention: Active Ingredients 155
The Crucible of Transformation 160
Suggestions for Compassion Fatigue Prevention and Resiliency............. 161
Conclusion 162

References 167

Appendices... 173
Appendix 1: Self-Regulation... 175
Appendix 2: Pinnacle Exercises 178
Appendix 3: Reactive to Intentional Worksheet 186
Appendix 4: Training Opportunities 187

Introduction
Trauma Practice: Tools for Stabilization and Recovery

*If you are perfect you don't need to learn anything
and if you don't need to learn anything, you wouldn't need to be a teacher.*
Stuart Wilde, *The Secrets of Life (1990)*

Purpose of This Book

This book is written for the trained clinician and the novice-in-training as a means of enhancing skilled application of Cognitive Behavioral Therapy (CBT) as trauma therapy. The term *Trauma Practice* has been conceptualized after many years of reflection of the trauma work and training experiences that the authors have encountered. It has become clear to us that a practical approach is needed for practitioners who apply themselves in the field of trauma treatment. Recent books and current research on CBT for trauma stabilization and recovery are focused more on outcome rather than application and we believe a practical "how-to" text is required. In addition, this text draws upon the development and implementation of many trauma-training programs that have been ongoing since the fall of 1997 through the Traumatology Institute. We have been training students in trauma recovery within this CBT framework and have found both a great need and a warm response to this very practical approach.

This book will provide both the novice and advanced trauma therapist with much of the knowledge and skills necessary to begin utilizing CBT in their treatment of trauma survivors. In addition to presenting a foundational understanding of the theoretical tenets of CBT, this book will also provide step-by-step explanations in many of the most popular and effective techniques of CBT. Some of these techniques include: Trigger List Development, Breath Training, Systematic Desensitization, Exposure Therapy, Story-Telling-Approaches Assertiveness Training, and Relaxation Training. The book is packed with practical approaches that we have used with our clients for many years. In this updated edition, we have replaced some less useful approaches with interventions that have proven more effective with clients and students of the Traumatology Institute.

The materials in this book are organized and presented from the perspective of the Tri-Phasic Model (Herman, 1992) for the treatment of trauma. In 2000, the International Society for Traumatic Stress Studies adopted Herman's Tri-Phasic Model as the standard of care for clinicians working with clients diagnosed with posttraumatic stress disorder (ISTSS, 2000).

These three phases of treatment – (1) Safety and Stabilization, (2) Trauma Memory Processing, and (3) Reconnection are thoroughly explored and become the organizing structure for this text. Specific treatment goals and techniques are offered for each of these three phases of treatment making this text a "hands-on" reference and guidebook for clinicians as they navigate through the potentially difficult treatment trajectory with clients who have survived trauma.

The authors wish to make a clear statement that this book is only a guidebook and does not substitute for training and supervised practice necessary to integrate these principles and techniques into practice. The authors have presented the materials found in this book in a two-day training program followed by a 20-hour supervised practicum through the Traumatology Institute (Canada) and Compassion Unlimited. Please see Appendix 4 for more information on these training courses. Training is now available online at http://www.ticlearn.com for those individuals who do not have direct access to face-to-face training programs or the opportunity to bring institute trainers to their locations. We believe that proper training and supervision is required to safely and successfully integrate these powerful techniques into practice with trauma survivors. We offer these principles and techniques based upon the belief that the primary responsibility of the clinician is to "*above all else, do no harm*." While persons suffering with posttraumatic stress have demonstrated their strength and resiliency by having survived some of the most painful and heinous experiences known to mankind, it is possible for the well-intended but untrained therapist to engage in treatment with survivors that can actually retraumatize their clients, thus resulting in failed treatment and rendering future treatment even more difficult and painful for the survivor.

Further complicating trauma care is the very real element of personality changes that establish themselves rigidly over time – forming interpersonal skills from a reactive position developed to keep one out of harm's way. Trauma survivors may have developed concurrent personality disorders and resulting behaviors that may have been useful at the time of the trauma but no longer serve the individual well. Although as clinicians we may aid our clients to resolve the traumatic memories, harness improved self-care skills and establish systems for reconnecting with meaningful community and activities, our clients may then have to tackle the personality structures that no longer work for them once trauma is extinguished.

Self-of-the-Therapist

In Friedman's (1996) landmark article entitled "PTSD Diagnosis and Treatment for Mental Health Clinicians," he argues strongly that the development and maintenance of the "self-of-the-therapist" may be one of the most important aspects of treatment with traumatized individuals. We have found, in our own practices and in our training programs, that the ability to develop and maintain a nonanxious presence while working with trauma survivors is a key ingredient to successful treatment outcomes and in maximizing the resiliency of the therapist.

Confronting traumatic material is painful and can be debilitating for the therapist. Many of the techniques presented in this text involve, in one way or another, the confrontation and narration of the traumatic experiences by the trauma survivor with support and guidance from the therapist. It is theorized that the ability of the trauma survivor to access, confront, and self-regulate while narrating traumatic experiences may be one of the active ingredients to the resolution of traumatic stress. The ability of the therapist to elicit, assist and self-regulate while the survivor struggles through these narrations is, in our opinion, an a priori requirement for effective treatment. Indeed, we have all worked with posttraumatic clients who have "failed" in previous therapy attempts because they were unable to complete these narratives with their therapists. We believe that a courageous, optimistic, and nonanxious approach, tempered with safety and pacing, to be the key to rapid amelioration of traumatic stress symptoms.

In our training programs, we work diligently toward helping therapists develop the capacity for self-regulation and the maintenance of a nonanxious presence. Recent research demonstrates that high levels of anxiety can diminish cognitive and motor functioning (Sapolsky, 1997; Scaer, 2001). This diminished capacity may account for some of the symptoms associated with traumatic stress. It may also point toward some of the difficulties encountered by therapists who work with clients who suffer from traumatic stress. Compassion fatigue (Figley, 1995, 2002) has recently become an important focus for therapists working with traumatic stress. We have included, as part of this text, a chapter written to help the trauma therapist understand the potential effects of working with trauma survivors. This chapter includes strategies for developing resiliency toward and prevention of the possible deleterious effects of helping. In addition, this chapter provides a model for the maturation of caregiving skills we believe to be important for the provision of consistently effective treatment to trauma survivors and the maintenance of quality of life for the trauma therapist.

Core Objectives

Upon completion of this book readers will be
- aware of the underlying principles of Behavioral, Cognitive, and Cognitive Behavioral Therapy that are reported to lead to the resolution of posttraumatic stress symptoms;

Introduction

- aware of the psychophysiology of posttraumatic stress;
- aware of how to apply Cognitive Behavioral Therapy toward the fulfillment of specific criteria in each of the three phases of the Tri-Phasic Model of treatment with trauma survivors;
- able to apply effective trauma stabilization and resolution interventions that best fit the unique requirements of any survivor;
- able to utilize many different Cognitive Behavioral Therapy techniques to help trauma survivors resolve the effects of their trauma memories and posttraumatic symptoms;
- able to utilize Cognitive Behavioral Therapy techniques to assist trauma survivors in developing more satisfying lifestyles in the present.

Book Description

CBT is one of the most researched and most effective treatments for posttraumatic stress disorder (PTSD) and we believe that all skilled traumatologists should have at least rudimentary understanding and skills in this important area of treatment. This book will focus upon the utilization of the principle of *reciprocal inhibition* (exposure + relaxation) as a core knowledge and skill that readers will acquire following a thorough reading and integration of the materials covered in this book. Nearly all of CBT is organized around this principle and we believe it can be found in most *effective* treatments of posttraumatic stress.

This book will begin with a brief outline of the history and the theoretical underpinnings of CBT. A brief discussion of possible physiological pathways to account for the identified behavioral phenomena will be included. This will be followed by an introduction to Herman's (1992) Tri-Phasic Model for the treatment of posttraumatic conditions. A thorough exploration of the *Safety and Stabilization* phase of treatment with an opportunity to practice and learn several skills for use in this aspect of treatment will follow.

After the reader has learned the skills necessary for the essential development of safety and stabilization with their clients, the book will focus on techniques useful for the successful resolution of traumatic memories in the Trauma Memory Processing phase of treatment. Readers will learn several specific CBT techniques for assisting their clients with accessing, confronting, and resolving their traumatic memories. These techniques will be presented in a step-by-step process with the goal of skills development. We hope this text will provide readers with a comfort level that will allow them to begin using these interventions in their service to trauma survivors.

The final area of this book, Reconnection, will focus on developing skills to assist trauma survivors in resolving the residual sequelae from their traumas. Often times, even after a survivor has successfully resolved a trauma memory, symptoms such as survivor guilt, distorted and self-critical thinking styles, relational dysfunction, addiction, or painful affect remain unresolved. This last phase of treatment is focused on helping the trauma survivor reconnect with themselves, their families, and loved ones in the present and to their goals for the future. Several CBT techniques will be presented to the reader for their use in helping their clients navigate successfully through this important phase of treatment.

With the completion of this book, the reader will have gained sufficient knowledge and skills to integrate the principles and techniques of CBT into their practice with survivors of trauma.

Supportive Texts and Other Recommended Readings

1. Herman, J. (1992). *Trauma and recovery.* New York: Basic Books.
2. Follette, V. M., Ruzek, J. I., & Abueg, F. R. (1998). *Cognitive-behavioral therapies for trauma.* New York: Guilford Press.
3. Rothbaum, B. O., Meadows, E. A., Resick, P., & Foy, D. (2000). Cognitive-behavioral therapy. In E. B. Foa, T. M. Keene, & M. J. Friedman (Eds.), *Effective treatment for PTSD* (pp. 60 – 83). New York: Guilford Press.
4. Seligman, M. (2002). *Authentic happiness.* New York: Free Press.

Section 1
Foundations of the Trauma Practice Model

For fast-acting relief from stress, try slowing down.
Lily Tomlin, American actress & comedienne

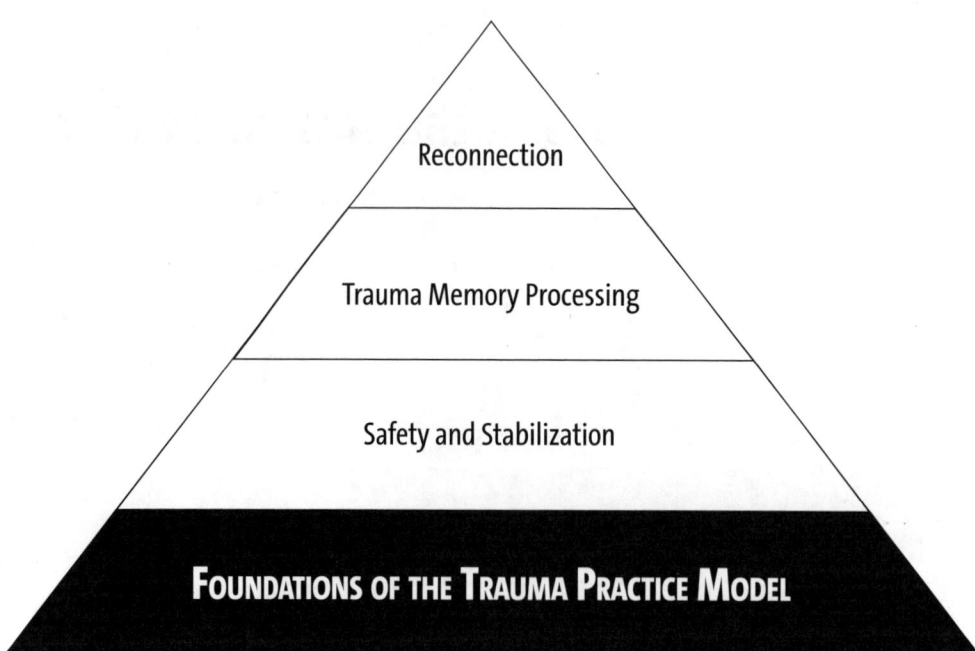

1. **Behavioral Therapy**
2. **Cognitive Therapy**
3. **Cognitive-Behavioral Therapy**
4. **Cognitive-Behavioral Therapy Research**
    Expert Guidelines
    The International Society for Traumatic Stress Studies (ISTSS) Practice Guidelines
5. **Psychophysiology of Trauma**
6. **Tri-Phasic Model**
    Safety and Stabilization
    Trauma Memory Processing
    Reconnection
7. **Necessary Ingredients – Treatment Codes (R, RE, CR)**
8. **Body, Cognition, Behavior, and Emotion/Relation**
9. **Posttrauma Response**

> Section 1 provides some of the current theories explaining both the cognitive and physiological underpinnings of the symptoms and successful interventions for the treatment of trauma. The symptoms that manifest from trauma are natural and normal sequelae to exposure to extraordinary events. Understanding the mechanism by which these occur will provide a much better ability to understand the variety of symptoms seen in practice. Understanding how the interventions are logically linked to the mechanism by which symptoms occur should provide a better ability to utilize the techniques presented and increase confidence in their effectiveness with clients. This understanding will help in the creation of on-the-spot interventions to also address the immediate needs of clients.

1. Behavioral Therapy

The origins of many current practices used to treat posttraumatic stress disorder (PTSD) and other posttraumatic conditions can be traced to a developmental history that includes Behavioral Therapy (BT). This is because BT, with its roots in classical and operant conditioning (i.e., Pavlov and Skinner), demonstrated a good outcome in addressing problems associated with fear and anxiety. It is interesting to note that practitioners of strict BT were uninterested in the events that occurred inside the minds of their clients. This was considered a black box that was not relevant to the outcome of behavioral interventions. A practitioner of pure BT was concerned primarily with the observable and manifest occurrences (or behaviors) in the lives of their clients and the specific antecedents that elicited those behaviors. They were not interested in what one thought of the events or how one interpreted or gave meaning to the events.

From the perspective of BT, the symptoms of posttraumatic stress occur in a two-step process that involves first classical conditioning and then operant conditioning. These two theories of "conditioning" explain why certain behaviors (in this case, symptoms of trauma) are likely to reoccur. In the 1890s to early 1900s, Pavlov investigated gastric function in dogs and reflex responses that led eventually to his theory of classical conditioning. He was awarded the Nobel Prize for this research in 1904. In classical conditioning, an unconditioned stimulus (UCS) such as meat powder is presented to an animal and it elicits salivation. This is a normal reaction to food and is called the *unconditioned response* (UCR). When the meat powder is paired with another (conditioned) stimulus (CS) such as a bell, time after time, eventually the bell will also elicit salivation. So although the bell is at first just peripheral sensory information to the meat powder, it is eventually associated as a signal that meat powder is present and elicits the physiological response of salivating, which is now called the *conditioned response* (CR). To unhook this response of salivation to the sound of the bell is called *extinguishing the behavior*. This involves presenting the bell many times without the associated meat powder. Eventually the bell no longer produces salivation.

To see an interactive example of how this works, visit http://nobelprize.org/educational_games/medicine/pavlov/

Operant conditioning suggests another mechanism to explain behaviors. In operant conditioning, the subject operates on the environment by performing behaviors. If the behaviors result in a favorable outcome (i.e., are reinforced), the subject is more likely to perform those behaviors again. Reinforcement of favorable outcomes might include actually getting something for the behavior (e.g., a pellet of food, a smile, etc.) or removing a noxious condition (e.g., a blaring noise or anxiety). The first is called *positive reinforcement* and the second is called *negative reinforcement*. Either form of reinforcement make behaviors more likely to occur. In operant conditioning, one way to make behaviors less likely to occur is to remove all reinforcement for the behaviors.

In the case of PTSD, the first form of conditioning that occurs is classical. In this instance, a traumatic event (the UCS) produces fear/anxiety/arousal (the UCR). This is a normal reaction to trauma, and it is a very powerful response associated with the survival mechanism. The brain is hardwired to attend to all information associated with survival and registers much of the sensory information peripheral to the traumatic event. Like the bell in Pavlov's experiments, this peripheral sensory information is the CS (i.e., all the sensory input peripheral to the traumatic event). However, unlike Pavlov's bell, which takes many pairings of the bell and meat powder to produce salivation, the association of the UCS/CS (traumatic event/all other sensory information) to fear/anxiety/arousal happens instantly. This is an example of one-trial learning. From that time forward, any time the CS (any sensory information that was associated with the original event) occurs, a CR (fear/anxiety/arousal) can potentially occur. This becomes problematic when, subsequent to a seemingly random sensory experience, this fear/anxiety/arousal response occurs. The brain has no specific event to associate to the fear response and begins to generalize it to more normal events not originally associated with the traumatic event. This makes the symptom picture seem very complex.

A simple example of this would be the anxiety associated with an automobile accident. The accident itself is the UCS, which generates a considerable amount of fear and anxiety (the UCR). For illustration purposes, say the accident occurred in heavy traffic with a considerable amount of exhaust fumes in the air, at a stop light, at dusk. These would be considered the conditioned sensory stimuli (CS). If the accident resulted in a severe response, these conditioned stimuli (fumes, stop lights, and dusk) might then produce the fear and anxiety associated with the original accident, even when there is no current threat of accident. The fear and anxiety produced by the conditioned stimuli are now referred to as the CR. Now, as exposure to traffic, exhaust fumes, stop lights, and dusk occur, the individual can be retriggered to the traumatic memory and associated physiological, behavioral, and emotional responses associated with the accident itself. Other sensory information can also generalize to the accident and become associated with the anxiety. For instance, the driving anxiety may recur in a different vehicle under new circumstances that do not include any dangerous events but illicit feelings of fear and emotional distress. The different vehicle, daylight hours, and driving in general are all potentially added to the list of conditioned stimuli and may subsequently evoke anxiety as well.

The problematic behaviors associated with PTSD, such as avoidance, social isolation, anxiety-provoked reactions (e.g., anger, startle response), self-medication through substance abuse, etc. are behaviors that are meant to reduce the anxiety associated with the event (or subsequently associated events). When the fear/anxiety/arousal response occurs, the individual performs behaviors meant to help alleviate the anxiety. These behaviors are maintained through an operant conditioning model, where the anxiety and arousal brought about by the conditioned stimuli are reduced by the problematic behavior. The behaviors are negatively reinforced and, thus, more likely to occur.

To continue with our accident example, the person who had the accident may begin to experience anxiety in heavy traffic, and/or when smelling exhaust fumes, and/or at stop lights, and/or at dusk while driving. To avoid this anxiety, this person may cease driving in any or all of the above conditions. When the person stops driving, the anxiety decreases. From the operant conditioning model, a noxious stimulus has been removed. This is negative reinforcement and the behavior of stopping, or even not venturing out, will be more likely to occur.

Figure 1 is a simple diagram of the first step in the creation of posttraumatic stress. This is the classical conditioning of the fear/anxiety/arousal response.

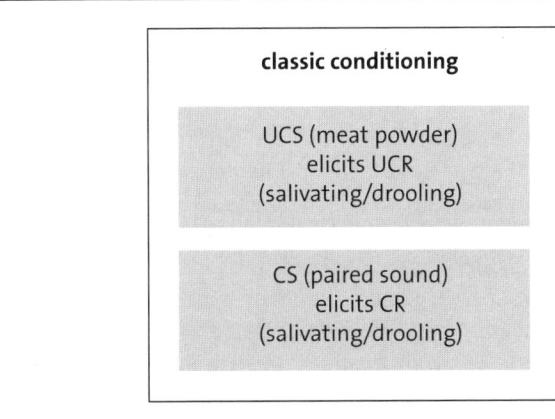
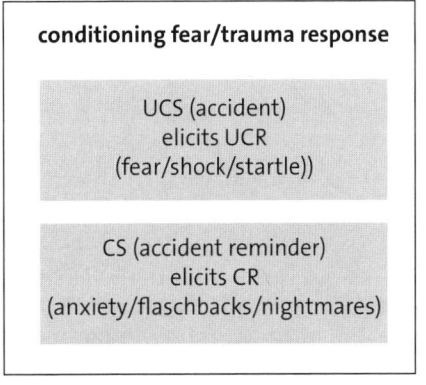

Figure 1. Classical conditioning of the fear/anxiety/arousal response.

> **Conditioned Response**
>
> = Fear/anxiety/arousal manifested through intrusive symptoms (i.e., nightmares, flashbacks)
>
> ↓
>
> **New Behaviors**
>
> Problematic behaviors performed in attempt to reduce fear/anxiety/arousal
>
> ↓
>
> **Reinforcement of New Behaviors**
>
> Anxienty reduced negatively, reinforcing problematic behaviors, making them more likely to occur

Figure 2. Operant conditioning: Problematic behavior is reinforced by removal of fear/anxiety/arousal.

In this simple learning theory model (Mower, 1960), the traumatic event (UCS) produces a fear response (UCR) and when the survivor experiences stimuli that have come to be associated with the event (CS), the fear returns to plague the survivor in the form of intrusive symptoms (e.g., nightmares and flashbacks) and arousal symptoms taking the form of rapid heart rate, shallow breathing, muscle tension, etc. (CR).

The second step explains the manifestation and maintenance of many of the problematic behaviors associated with posttraumatic stress such as avoidance, substance abuse, anger, etc. This step is an example of operant conditioning wherein a problematic behavior is reinforced by the removal of fear/anxiety/arousal (see Figure 2).

In other words, as the survivor is continually confronted with this fear, they begin to develop behaviors to help alleviate the arousal and anxiety associated with the stimuli (CS). These behaviors are likely to include avoidance of the objects, people, and events that trigger remembrances of the traumatic event and the negative emotions associated with them. The behaviors may also include those meant to dull the intensity of the emotions such as substance use or emotional withdrawal. From the BT perspective, this ever-widening circle of arousal and avoidance is thought to be the essence of PTSD.

The actual practice of BT involves carrying out a "functional analysis" of the survivor's environment to help identify stimuli and reinforcers that elicit and maintain problematic behaviors. However, the essence of the resolution of PTSD using BT requires that the survivor begin to confront, rather than avoid, the traumatic memory and the triggers associated with the trauma. This confrontation may be of the actual memory and/or the triggers associated with the trauma. The survivor is given skills to help him/her address the fear/anxiety/arousal and challenged to remain engaged in these confrontation/exposure situations until the fear diminishes and symptoms are, ultimately, extinguished.

For the trauma survivor, confronting their memories of abuse, horror, terror, and pain are often like riding a dangerously bucking bronco. The memories elicit the fear/anxiety/arousal associated with the original event and create a huge disincentive to do the work. It is a challenging process that demands skill, patience, and assistance from both the client and the therapist. Nonetheless, just as the horse adjusts to the rider and the dog stops salivating over time (when a bell is rung and meat powder is never produced), a trauma survivor can also learn to experience a trauma memory without eliciting the response of fear/anxiety/arousal. The behavioral therapist assists the trauma survivor by structuring the treatment process in a way that allows them to gain mastery of this response.

In 1958, Joseph Wolpe, a behavioral therapist and researcher, developed the theory of reciprocal inhibition (Wolpe, 1958) to explain and direct the treatment of anxiety and phobia symptoms. The theory of reciprocal inhibition holds that when exposure to an anxiety-provoking stimulus is paired with the relaxation response (i.e., the individual is able to keep the muscles in their body relaxed) and the client is able to maintain this relaxation, then the conditioned response to the fear-provoking stimulus is extinguished (see Figure 3). There are sound physiological reasons to explain the one-trial learning of classical conditioning and why reciprocal inhibition works that will be discussed more fully in the Psychophysiology of Trauma section.

Reciprocal inhibition, the pairing of exposure and relaxation, is at the heart of all BT with symptoms of anxiety. Some BTs (e.g., *in vivo* exposure or flooding) begin with exposure and push their way through the anxiety, hopefully to a point where the client is relaxed in the face of exposure. However, these techniques have the potential of retraumatizing the client if the individual is not able to fully maintain relaxation throughout the exposure exercise and as well if there is insufficient time to resolve or habituate to the trauma memory, leaving the trauma memory work incomplete. It is not until relaxation occurs in the face of exposure that symptoms subside. It is our opinion that relaxation is a necessary ingredient to symptom resolution and better learned before and experienced during exposure than experienced after the process of being overwhelmed by anxiety. Thus, we identify reciprocal inhibition as a "necessary ingredient" in effective treatments of PTSD. Most of the learning involved in this book will focus on teaching you, the reader, skilled application and utilization of reciprocal inhibition. You will learn techniques to help clients approach and confront their traumatic material. You will also learn techniques for assisting them in developing and maintaining the relaxation response during this exposure. The ability to assist the client in maximal attenuation of this process, also know as *titration*, can rapidly accelerate the treatment of PTSD and is the artful skill of the traumatologist.

Present-day practitioners of strict BT are still primarily interested in behaviors and a functional analysis of the specific life occurrences that elicit dysfunctional behaviors. However, as you might expect, they have come to believe that the mind may mediate some of these events. While they still help their clients focus on their problematic behaviors (or failure to practice positive behaviors) and assist them with stopping or eradicating these problematic behaviors and/or learning and practicing new, more fulfilling behaviors (Follette, Ruzek, & Abueg, 1998), some of these interventions are, now, decidedly cognitive.

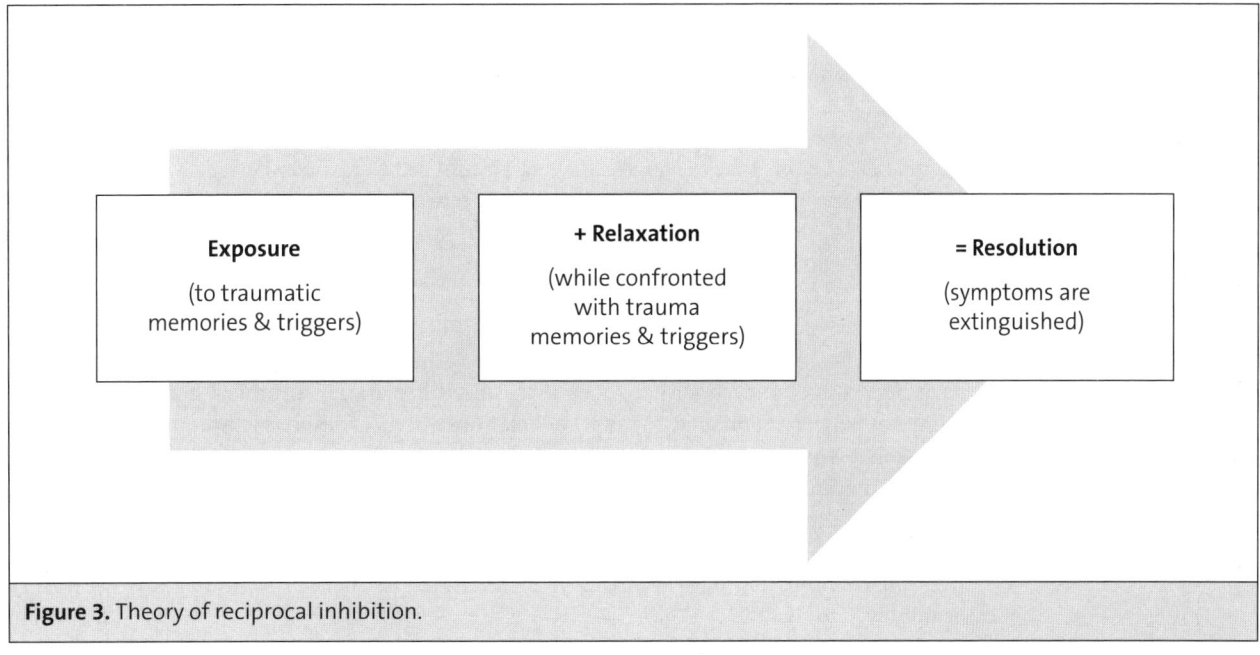

Figure 3. Theory of reciprocal inhibition.

The BT process known as Direct Therapeutic Exposure, which was commonly utilized with Vietnam veterans, is an example of this procedure. In this process, a functional analysis of the client's life is performed wherein a number of factors are assessed. These include, but are not limited to, safety, secondary gain, resources, other life traumas, triggers, and reinforcers. Target behaviors are also identified. Then, a considerable amount of psychoeducation occurs. The client is taught relaxation techniques, learns coping skills, is specifically taught the two-step process of symptom generation to normalize the experience, and has the process of exposure in therapy explained. After the client has demonstrated adequate stabilization, they begin the process of remembering what happened with full affect. The client is encouraged to stay with the process until the anxiety lessens. This may take repeating the memory process several times. Once they have finished, the therapist assists in returning them to a state of relaxation. The therapist then processes the information, helping the client create new meanings and beliefs about the experience. In other words, they begin the process of cognitive restructuring. The exciting part of this work is seeing client transformation through exposure and then habituation resulting in extinction of the trigger or the traumatic memory. When it comes to extinction of traumatic memories, the result is a lessening of reactivity when exposed to trauma reminders in the future. Although this process is explained above, the Trauma Practice approach allows for alternative methods to achieve the desired outcome.

2. Cognitive Therapy

In the 1960s and early 1970s, and, many would say, in reaction to BT's clinically sterile fascination with only manifest behaviors, clinical and research psychologists became progressively more interested in what was happening *inside* the client who was suffering with symptoms of anxiety and depression. Scientists like Ellis (Ellis & Harper, 1961) and Beck (1967, 1976) began to investigate the importance of a client's thoughts, and the meanings, beliefs, and interpretations they attached to events for both the understanding and treatment of psychological disorders and their symptoms.

A cognitive therapist would be quick to point out that not everyone who experiences the same traumatic event develops posttraumatic symptoms and those who do have a vast array of different consequences from the same event. From the perspective of Cognitive Therapy (CT), this difference was due to the survivor's beliefs, meanings, interpretations, and other *internal* events and reactions to the traumatic experience. Cognitive therapists believe that certain (traumatic) events, especially during developmental periods, can result in the entire belief system, or schema, becoming distorted. These distorted schemas continue to shape and misshape the world for many trauma survivors. Treatment is oriented toward identifying the distorted beliefs that survivors attach to painful or traumatic experiences and helping the survivor renegotiate these beliefs and meanings toward more healthy and adaptive ones. This process of assisting a client in changing or rescripting their distorted thoughts of themselves and their world is called *cognitive restructuring*.

A common example of this is a client who had been molested in childhood. Because her abuser used words like "sexy" and "pretty" during the abuse, she came to believe that it must have been something about her looks that caused her abuser to molest her. To insure that it did not happen again, she began to overeat obsessively, in the mistaken belief that being overweight would make her less "sexy" and protect her from being molested again. As years pass she may no longer remember the first thought of making herself less attractive. However, subsequent attempts to lose weight are not only unsuccessful, they result in a considerable increase in anxiety. Treatment would involve identifying the distorted belief about why she was abused in the first place and help in restructuring her belief system to allow her a more healthy way to be safe.

Cognitive therapists assist clients first in identifying their distorted thoughts and beliefs and then help them substitute new, more satisfying beliefs. Techniques like Thought Stopping, Positive Affirmations, Rehearsal, and the Triple Column Technique (Burns, 1980) are all frequently utilized in CT to assist the client in shifting these thinking patterns.

There exists a debate among cognitive therapists about whether or not it is important to gain insight and understanding as to the causes and events that gave rise to distorted thought patterns. Some believe that focusing treatment energy and resources on assisting the client in developing more satisfying beliefs, thoughts, and lifestyle in the present is the most crucial ingredient to therapy. Others believe this minimizes the importance of revisiting the traumatic events and the meanings ascribed to them; such therapists spend more time identifying the specific distorted thoughts that arise from the events.

For reasons discussed shortly, we believe the value of helping the trauma survivor develop more satisfactory living skills in the present, including the ability to utilize positive thinking and beliefs, is a necessary ingredient for symptom resolution and should be included in any treatment of trauma. We will utilize many techniques drawn from CT to teach methods for assisting the trauma survivor in developing this present-day stabilization and satisfaction. However, we will also utilize CT techniques to teach readers of this book to assist trauma survivors in confronting and resolving their traumatic memories. These procedures involve a combination of both CT (helping the survivor resolve their thoughts and meanings about the trauma, themselves, and the world) with the techniques of BT (helping the trauma survivor confront and resolve the traumatic memory using reciprocal inhibition). This combination results in a powerful collection of techniques known as *Cognitive Behavioral Therapy* (CBT) and is the focus of this book.

3. Cognitive-Behavioral Therapy

CBT is probably the most utilized, most researched, and most consistently effective treatment for the symptoms of posttraumatic stress currently used by clinicians who treat trauma survivors (Foa & Meadows, 1997). CBT combines the aspects of BT and CT, so it includes both explicit and observable, as well as the implicit and internal behaviors. Many writers have acknowledged the "cognitivization" of BT over recent years and a blurring of boundaries between CT, BT, and CBT.

Follette, Ruzek, and Abueg (1998) wrote:
> "As the field of behavioral therapy has evolved, it has generated a large number of both broad and specific theories that sometimes compliment one another and sometime compete for explanatory relevance. Indeed, there has been much debate about whether such a range of theoretical formulations can or should be accommodated under a single rubric of "behavioral therapy" or "cognitive-behavioral therapy," when alternative formulations sometimes do violence to the core assumptions and conceptual underpinnings of one another. With the growth in trauma-related cognitive-behavioral research and treatment, these same controversies are present. However, we believe there is some movement toward rapprochement among these differing perspectives." (pp. 4–5).

For the purposes of this book, we will integrate the principles and techniques of BT and CT together and identify these principles and techniques as CBT.

What we think is absolutely essential in how we live our lives. It is a large part in the determining factor of why some individuals experience PTSD after an event and others do not.

Conclusions or assumptions are often at the root of PTSD and at times if we can make good sense of an event or challenge distorted cognitions (beliefs) we may be able to change old beliefs, such as "I am never safe" to "I am safe in this moment right now!"

Doing good clinical trauma therapy means addressing the distorting cognitions that are negatively impacting the client's life, limiting their activities, outlets, and life pleasures. These include:
1. identifying distorted beliefs;
2. identifying the root of the distortion (when did the belief first surface? what happened at that time?);
3. extinguishing the old belief (often through various exposure and/or challenging exercises);
4. developing new more adaptive and intentional schemas or belief systems (e.g., I am doing my best).

4. Cognitive-Behavioral Therapy Research

Expert Guidelines

There are a considerable number of CBT techniques available to address the symptoms of PTSD. Choosing which is the most appropriate might seem confusing. When selecting the most appropriate therapeutic intervention to utilize with specific client groups it is important to look to both research *and* expert consensus to guide us. Although research can provide us with information about the factors associated with recovery, there are several reasons why the use of expert guidelines can also be useful in your day-to-day practice.

First, research does not always generalize easily into clinical practice and research studies often fail to reflect the complexities of the cases that we must address in our caseload. Second, systematic studies frequently fail to answer all the questions that arise in clinical practice in a comprehensive and effective manner. Third, research can be a tedious and time-consuming practice that does not move as quickly as meaningful and efficacious clinical innovation. This does not mean we discard the excellent research that highlights strong clinical methodology but that we supplement it with the best methods endorsed by expert consensus. This type of "research in motion" is certainly the lifeblood of all new and useful approaches.

One source of expert guidelines we can consider is the "Expert Consensus Guidelines Series: Treatment of Posttraumatic Stress Disorder" (Foa, Davidson, & Frances, 1999). This is a series in which 52 psychotherapy experts make recommendations based on their clinical experience and 57 medication experts make recommendations based on their experience treating PTSD. For further elucidation please refer directly to this supplemental journal, pp. 6–7.

The International Society for Traumatic Stress Studies (ISTSS) Practice Guidelines

CBT is the most widely researched treatment approach identified in the literature. In *Effective Treatments for PTSD* (Foa, Keane, & Friedman, 2000), chapter 4 contains a literature review of current CBT research (Rothbaum et al., 2000). The focus of this review addresses a number of brief CBT interventions. These include: Exposure Therapy (ET); Systematic Desensitization (SD); Stress Inoculation Training (SIT); Cognitive Processing Therapy (CPT); Cognitive Therapy (CT); Assertiveness Training (AT); Biofeedback (BIO); Relaxation Training (Relax), and various combinations of those listed above.

Table 1. Preferred psychotherapy techniques for different PTSD target symptoms		
Most prominent symptom	**Recommended techniques**	**Also consider**
Intrusive thoughts	Exposure Therapy	Cognitive Therapy Anxiety Management Psychoeducation Play Therapy for Children
Flashbacks	Exposure Therapy	Anxiety Management Cognitive Therapy Psychoeducation
Trauma-related fears, panic, & avoidance	Exposure Therapy Cognitive Therapy Anxiety Management	Psychoeducation Play Therapy for Children
Numbing/detachment from others/loss of interest	Cognitive Therapy	Psychoeducation Exposure Therapy
Irritability/angry outbursts	Cognitive Therapy Anxiety Management	Psychoeducation Exposure Therapy
Guilt/shame	Cognitive Therapy	Psychoeducation Play Therapy for Children
General Anxiety (hyperarousal, hypervigilance, startle)	Anxiety Management Exposure Therapy	Cognitive Therapy Psychoeducation Play Therapy for Children
Sleep disturbances	Anxiety Management	Exposure Therapy Cognitive Therapy Psychoeducation
Difficulty concentrating	Anxiety Management	Cognitive Therapy Psychoeducation

From: Foa, E. B., Davidson, J. R. T., & Frances, A. The Expert Consensus Guideline Series: Treatment of Posttraumatic Stress Disorder. *The Journal of Clinical Psychiatry 1999; 60:15.* Copyright 1999 Physicians Postgraduate Press. Adapted/reprinted by permission.

Table 2. Selecting psychotherapy techniques based on effectiveness, safety, acceptability, and speed of action		
Technical approach	**Recommended techniques**	**Also consider**
Most-effective techniques	Exposure Therapy Cognitive Therapy	Anxiety Management
Quickest-acting techniques	Exposure Therapy	Anxiety Management Cognitive Therapy Psychoeducation
Techniques preferred across all types of trauma	Cognitive Therapy Exposure Therapy Anxiety Management	Psychoeducation
Safest techniques	Anxiety Management Psychoeducation Cognitive Therapy	Play Therapy for Children Exposure Therapy
Most-acceptable techniques	Psychoeducation Cognitive Therapy Anxiety Management	Play Therapy for Children

From: Foa, E. B., Davidson, J. R. T., & Frances, A. The Expert Consensus Guideline Series: Treatment of Posttraumatic Stress Disorder. *The Journal of Clinical Psychiatry 1999; 60:17.* © 1999 Physicians Postgraduate Press. Adapted/reprinted by permission.

Table 3. CBT research synthesis

Intervention	Number of studies reviewed	AHCPR rating	Gold standards for clinical studies	Summary
ET	12	Level A (8 studies) Level B – (4 studies)	Mixed results. Several met all 7 standards while some met notably fewer.	"Compelling evidence ... quite effective" (p. 75).
SD	6	Level A through C Most B or lower	None met all 7 standards	Methodological problems and failed to receive strong research based support (p. 75).
SIT	4	Level A (2 studies) Level B – (2 "...")	Mixed results. Rigor of studies varies.	"Found SIT effective" (p. 76). Focus only on female sexual assault survivors.
CPT	1	Level B	Meets 4 of 7 standards.	"Effective" (p. 76). Modify to various trauma populations.
CT	3	Level A to C	Mixed results.	"CT ... effective in reducing ... symptoms" (p.76).
AT	1	Level B	Moderate adherence to 3 of 7 standards.	"Has not received strong support" (p. 77).
BIO & Relax	1	Level A	Meets 4 of 7 standards.	"BIO and Relax have not received support" (p. 77).

See Rothbaum et al., 2000.

Each of the many research studies reviewed were subsequently organized based on type of treatment, adherence to the Gold Standards Rating and the Agency for Health Care Policy and Research (AHCPR) ratings. These standards rate research based on a seven-point system that categorizes level of methodological rigor. Studies can be categorized as Level A – Very well controlled or methodologically rigorous; Level B – Less well controlled or moderately rigorous methodology; Level C or lower – Not well controlled or weak studies. The following table is a synthesis of this literature review (Rothbaum, et al., 2000).

It is clear that the CBT outcome results in this review are mixed. Nevertheless, CBT stands out in the literature as more efficacious than any other single approach in the psychological treatment of trauma. To understand this discrepancy, it is necessary to recall the limitations of research based on this review. First, we are always limited to the research currently available – methods may be clinically "effective" but not yet supported by research; second, studies available may have been conducted using poor methodologies; third, we cannot necessarily generalize the utility of a well-studied approach for one population based on another (e.g., Exposure Therapy for PTSD based on research for depressed married females). Therefore, it is useful to refer back to the expert guidelines discussed earlier. It is also important to recognize that some of the most effective approaches such as Exposure Therapy require a skilled practitioner to implement because the possibility of retriggering can occur if the client has not been adequately taught to initiate stabilization and self-care if symptoms become overwhelming.

5. Psychophysiology of Trauma

The hows and whys of posttraumatic stress, subsequent symptoms, and symptom resolution can be understood in relation to the events that occur in the brain during and after a traumatic event. What follows is a *brief* description of the sequence of events during and after a trauma. This information is extremely useful when educating survivors and explaining that their symptoms are natural responses to extreme events. For a more complete understanding of the neurological sequence involved in trauma, see Sapolsky, 1997; Scaer, 2006; van der Kolk, McFarlane, & Weisaeth, 1996; Rothschild, 2000; and Johnson, 2003.

When a person experiences a traumatic event, the information is registered in the brain along two pathways. The first and quickest path sends sensory information (e.g., scent, related objects, sounds, sights, etc.) to the amygdala, where a fear response is triggered and the information is cataloged as important for survival. From the amygdala, the information proceeds to other areas of the brain (i.e., the stria terminalis and the locus ceruleus) responsible for preparing the body for flight or fight and a subsystem of the autonomic nervous system (the sympathetic nervous system) is activated. The information is eventually stored in the hippocampus as a memory important for survival. Thereafter, anything that stimulates that sensory memory trace will also potentially stimulate the body to prepare for survival (fear/anxiety/arousal). In other words, when an individual is exposed to related cues to the memory (e.g., scent, related objects, sounds, sights, etc.) these sensory reminders reignite the associated strong feelings. The memory of the traumatic event itself may or may not be recalled. This can leave the individual feeling as if they are in danger but not necessarily knowing why.

This variability in memory can be understood by following the second pathway for information processing. This second and much longer path for the information proceeds through the thalamus, which routes sensory information to appropriate parts of the neocortex to be analyzed. This information is processed through various areas in the neocortex where language is used to organize and generate responses (a declarative memory is formed), associations to other information are made, and meaning is created. It is then routed to and stored in the hippocampus. The neocortex also contains inhibitory areas that are capable of inhibiting or turning down the survival/fear response generated by the information passed through the amygdala. In other words, the neocortex can potentially change the meaning of the original memory trace and alter or modulate the survival response.

Under conditions of extreme stress, the brain produces stress hormones such as cortisol that interfere with the consolidation of the information from the neocortex. This also interferes with the possible inhibitory responses that would ameliorate the anxiety of the survival response. Memories that are formed under conditions of trauma often become fragmented. They remain out of context and are thus left unincorporated and unassociated with other memories. The result is that, whenever the memory trace is stimulated, the body reverts to survival mode, which is experienced as anxiety. Because the traumatic memories are often unconsolidated, it is sometimes difficult for a survivor to make the link between earlier traumatic experiences and the current feeling of anxiety. The individual then begins to perform behaviors to relieve the anxiety. If these behaviors work to relieve the anxiety (i.e., remove a noxious condition), they are negatively reinforced to occur again.

These information storage pathways account for the symptoms discussed in the previous example of the person who was involved in an accident. During this accident, a large number of sensory cues were recorded such as the smell of exhaust fumes, heavy traffic, and dim light. This sensory information is recorded in such a manner that, even without actually remembering the original accident, the person in the accident might find themselves becoming extremely anxious at the smell of exhaust fumes or being in heavy traffic at dusk. Because they do not actually remember the original event, they will try to make sense of their feelings using information from the current moment. This is often a confusing task, especially if there is nothing particularly threatening in the current moment. They may just assume they are having an "anxiety attack" and attribute it to a physiological problem. Or they may simply begin to perform behaviors to reduce their anxiety, such as self-medicating with drugs or alcohol or avoiding driving.

The initial neurological response of the brain is likely the mechanism by which the classical conditioning of the traumatic response is accomplished. In one-trial learning, the sensory stimuli are sent to the midbrain and recorded as a threat to survival. The brain attaches the emotions of fear and anxiety to these stimuli and prepares the body for flight or fight. Very little cognitive processing occurs at this stage because the neocortex has been flooded with cortisol and other corticosteroids that interfere with memory consolidation. The fact that memories are unconsolidated and unconnected results in the failure to normally resolve the fear/anxiety/arousal response. In other words, the brain has failed to unhook the sensory information from the fear/anxiety/arousal response. Later behaviors are operationally learned as a way to alleviate this fear/anxiety/arousal.

Subsequent stimulation of this memory trace will potentially reactivate the survival routines until the neocortex has been allowed to process the information and inhibit the response. Relaxation in the face of exposure facilitates access to neocortical functions (declarative memory, meaning generation, and anxiety inhibition). Recent research suggests that this may be mediated by a decrease in cortisol under conditions of relaxation (Benson, 1997; Luecken, Dausch, Gulla, Hong, & Compas, 2004; Mason, Giller, Kosten, & Harkness, 1988). Strictly behavioral interventions pair the memory trace with responses (relaxation, self-soothing) that are inconsistent with the survival mode (fear/anxiety/arousal), expanding the response set. Cognitive interventions specifically work to pair the memory trace with more fully processed (and hence more meaningful) information that has the ability to inhibit the survival response.

Recall the client who experienced an automobile accident. The sensory stimuli are sent to the midbrain and recorded as a threat to survival. The brain attaches the emotions of fear and anxiety to these stimuli and prepares the body for flight or fight. As expected, little cognitive processing occurs at this stage, and the neocortex becomes flooded with cortisol and other corticosteroids, essentially inhibiting the ability to consolidate and fully store memories. Future reminders of the memory will reignite the poorly stored memory trace of the event, resulting in survival strategies being engaged. Survival responses will continue to occur until neocortical processing of the traumatic memory has adequately allowed for restorage of the memory while concurrently extinguishing the emotional distress associated with the memory. An *in vivo* (onsite) behavioral intervention would teach relaxation techniques and then pair relaxation with the sensory stimulus. In this example, a client would be relaxed and then perhaps be taken into traffic or allowed to smell exhaust by the roadside until they become anxious. The client would then initiate relaxation exercises until the symptoms of anxiety begin to reduce. This can occur either *in vivo* or after departing from the anxiety-provoking situation. This might require many exposures until the client was no longer anxious in the presence of fumes or traffic. Cognitive interventions also require teaching relaxation techniques and reexperiencing the event. However, these would more likely involve the client intentionally remembering the traumatic event under conditions of relaxation rather than direct experience of traumatic stimuli. Initial sessions would involve discussions of memories peripheral to the actual trauma and subsequent beliefs about the event. Eventually, trauma reduction sessions would involve the direct memory of the event (again, under conditions of relaxation) and the ability to describe the event without anxiety. Finally, cognitive restructuring would address distorted beliefs and behaviors previously learned and used to keep safe.

Offering posttrauma care that addresses the impact of the trauma on our brain functioning requires that the clinician assist the client to slow down the reactivity ignited when the individual is exposed to trauma reminders that set off old emotions. It is the gap between exposure to trauma reminders and reactivity that opens the door to change. It is pausing in that gap with calm reflection that allows us inform and reform our reactivity, creating a new storage of the trauma memory associated with a more reflective and less reactive or emotionally strained response. Our goal in *Trauma Practice* is to find the route to retraining the brain along with the body, mind, and emotion.

6. Tri-Phasic Model

Judith Herman is a psychiatrist in the Boston area. She has worked extensively with trauma expert Bessel van der Kolk. Herman is the author of two books, *Father Daughter Incest* (1981) and *Trauma and Recovery* (1992), and numerous articles on the enduring effects of chronic trauma. *Trauma and Recovery* is considered a seminal work on the history and treatment of chronic Type II trauma. Herman conceives trauma recovery to proceed in three stages:
1. Safety and Stabilization;
2. Remembrance and Mourning, which we will now refer to as *Trauma Memory Processing*;
3. Reconnection.

Safety and Stabilization

The central task of recovery is safety. Victims of chronic trauma are betrayed both by their experiences as well as their own bodies. Their symptoms become the source of triggers that result in retraumatization. The clinician's primary goal is to help the client regain internal and external control. This is accomplished through careful diagnosis, education, and skills development. The safety section of this book is focused on skills development to aid the trauma survivor to practice self-soothe and self-care skills to increase emotional and behavioral stabilization. In cases where the client remains in an unsafe environment, plans to establish personal and practical safety remain the focus of treatment prior to delving into Trauma Memory Processing work. The overriding goal is to enable the client to make a gradual shift from "unpredictable danger to reliable safety" (p. 155), both in their environment and within themselves. Accomplishing this goal depends on the circumstances, as well as on the internal ability to cope with exposure to trauma memories; it may require days, weeks, or months to achieve.

Trauma Memory Processing

In the second phase of recovery, the client begins to work more deeply with exercises to process their trauma history, bringing unbearable memories to greater resolution. Because of the nature of traumatic memories, this process is rarely linear. Bits and pieces of the traumatic events emerge and can be processed. The objective is to create a space in which the client can safely work through traumatic events and begin to make sense of the devastating experiences that have shaped their life. The clinician's role is to "bear witness" to the client's experiences and help them find the fortitude to heal.

There are many excellent CBT techniques that fit well within the rubric of this stage of Trauma Memory Processing. In addition, there are newer approaches such as Eye Movement Desensitization and Reprocessing (EMDR), Time-Limited Trauma Therapy (TLTT), and Traumatic Incident Reduction (TIR); these approaches will not be covered in this book, but they certainly fit the CBT trauma therapy framework and warrant further exploration.

Reconnection

The final stage of recovery involves redefining oneself in the context of meaningful relationships and engagement in life activities. Trauma survivors gain closure on their experiences when they are able to see the things that happened to them with the knowledge that these events do not determine who they are. Trauma survivors are liberated by the conviction that, regardless of what else happens to them, they always have themselves. Many survivors are also sustained by an abiding faith in a higher power that they believe delivered them from oppressive terror. In many instances, survivors find a "mission" through which they can continue to heal and to grow. They may even end up helping others with similar histories of abuse and neglect. Successful resolution of the effects of trauma is a powerful testament to the indomitability of the human spirit. After Phase II of Trauma Practice is completed, personality that has been shaped through trauma must then be given the opportunity for new growth experiences that offer the hope of a widening circle of connections and the exploration of a broader range of interests.

7. Necessary Ingredients – Treatment Codes (R, RE, CR)

We believe there are three active and necessary ingredients for the effective treatment of trauma. These include relaxation and exposure (reciprocal inhibition) and cognitive restructuring. Note, however, that none of the ingredients by itself is sufficient to accomplish the task of recovery. Each of the techniques included in this book is intended to provide at least one of the three ingredients. Because the timing of the interventions is important as well, some of the techniques are most appropriate during the Safety and Stabilization phase, while others are more appropriate to the Trauma Memory Processing or Reconnection phases.

We will indicate which techniques provide which of the three ingredients with the following coding system:
R = relaxation, self-soothing
RE = relaxation and exposure
CR = cognitive restructuring

We chose to include a broad variety of interventions because different interventions will work more effectively with different clients, depending on their background and/or mode of experiencing. It is by no means an exhaustive list of interventions.

The type of intervention selected for each client is left to the creative discretion of the therapist. It is our hope that, with experience and an understanding of the necessary ingredients and process for trauma recovery, good therapists will be able to mix, mingle, and create interventions of their own to meet the specific needs of each client.

8. Body, Cognition, Behavior, and Emotion/Relation

Throughout this book you will notice that sections are broken down into Body, Cognition, Behavior, and Emotion/Relation. The reason for this is that we process events on many channels and sometimes it is necessary to recover both our ability to live peacefully in our Bodies (e.g., psychophysiology, heart rate, breathing); our Minds/Cognitions (e.g., thoughts, perceptions, and beliefs); our Behaviors (e.g., proactive vs. restricted); and our Emotions/Relations (e.g., range, depth, rationality, support level). With these elements in mind, we have made it our mission to seek out interventions that address recovery on all channels. By addressing different channels as needed, we gear our treatment to the client and thereby avoid "cookie cutter" methodology that limits our ability to truly treat the complexities so often common among those suffering from posttrauma syndromes.

9. Posttrauma Response

Based on the *Diagnostic and Statistical Manual of Mental Disorders,* Fourth Edition, Text Revision (*DSM-IV-TR*)(APA, 2000) diagnostic features, the most salient posttrauma elements result in the development of particular symptoms as a result of exposure to massive trauma in which one's personal health and well-being is threatened. The stressor is often identified as one that may lead to one's death or injury or to that of a person close to the individual (e.g., friend, family, colleague). There are six criteria that need to be met in part or whole to establish PTSD as a diagnosis. The PTSD diagnosis is based on the following criteria (APA, 2000):

- A1, personal involvement in a life-or-death event that is a threat to personal safety or that of friends, associates, or family;
- A2, the person responds to the stressor with horror, helplessness, or great fear;
- B, recurrent, intrusive mental reexperiencing of the trauma;
- C, avoidance of trauma-related cues and emotional numbing;
- D, hyperarousal;
- E, PTSD must be present for longer than one month; and
- F, the symptoms must be significant enough to impair functioning of life skills.

Other possible diagnoses to consider might include: Acute Stress Disorder; Generalized Anxiety Disorder; Major Depressive Disorder; Panic Disorder; Adjustment Disorder; Dissociative Disorders; or Dysthymia.

The wording of the diagnostic criterion for PTSD in the *DSM-IV-TR* recognizes that the individual's response to a traumatic event is equal in importance to the objective evaluation of the event itself and the degree to which it might be determined to be traumatic. By taking into account individual responses, we are able to begin to make sense of why some individuals become debilitated after experiencing a seemingly innocuous event, whereas others can spend long periods of time in the midst of heinous circumstances without developing negative effects.

To recap, key posttrauma symptoms include:
- feelings of horror, helplessness or fear;
- recurrent, intrusive reexperiencing of the traumatic event (e.g., nightmares, flashbacks, intrusive memory replay);
- avoidance of any trauma-related cues (e.g., places, people, or activities associated with the trauma or resulting in reminders of the trauma);
- anxious arousal (e.g., increase in heart rate and breathing, nervousness, fearfulness, agitation, easily ignited startle response); and
- impairment of life skills (e.g., ability to socialize, work, attend school, or manage family responsibilities)

Table 4. Features associated with posttrauma response

Alexithymia	Sadness and depression
Guilt over acts of commission or omission	Feelings of being overwhelmed
Survival guilt	Loss of assumptive world
Suicidal/homicidal ideation/behaviors	Behavioral reenactments
Disillusionment with authority	Self-destructive soothing behaviors
Feelings of hopelessness/helplessness	Somatization
Memory impairment and forgetfulness	Relationship problems

See Rothbaum et al. (2000).

In addition, there are two types of trauma that the traumatologist would benefit from differentiating at the beginning stage of treatment to assist in treatment planning.

Type I Trauma. An unexpected and discrete experience that overwhelms the individual's ability to cope with the stress, fear, threat, and/or horror of this event, leading to PTSD (e.g., motor vehicle accident, natural disaster). It is possible that the trauma might be in the form of witnessing an event (secondary traumatic stress). Treatment outcome tends to be achieved more rapidly than in Type II trauma if services are offered within a reasonable time (months rather than years) after onset of posttrauma symptoms.

Type II Trauma. Expected, but unavoidable, ongoing experience(s) that overwhelm the individual's ability to metabolize the event (e.g., childhood sexual abuse, combat trauma). This type of trauma is the origin of Disorders of Extreme Stress Not Otherwise Specified (DESNOS) and Dissociative Disorders.

Section 2
Safety and Stabilization

Your enemy is not well or healthy or strong and is unable to think straight or see straight because of her obsession with you ... no longer let this poor, weak creature have the power to upset you.
Susan Trott, *The Holy Man* (1995)

Reconnection

Trauma Memory Processing

SAFETY AND STABILIZATION

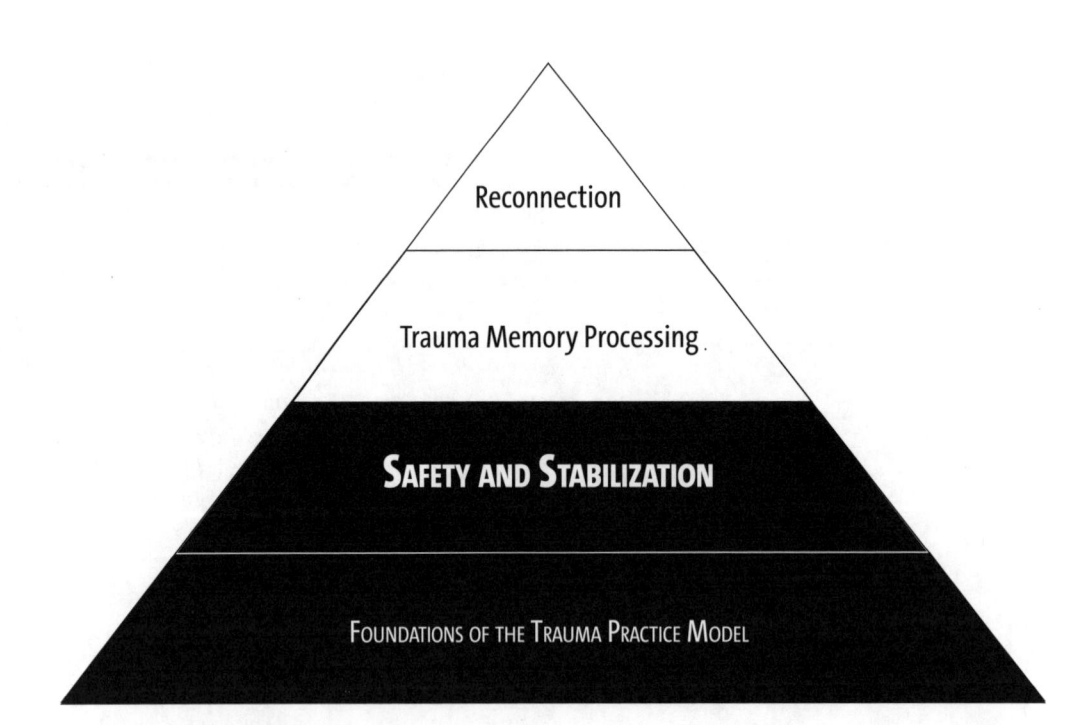

FOUNDATIONS OF THE TRAUMA PRACTICE MODEL

1. What Is Safety?
Minimum Criterion Required for Transition to Phase II Treatment

2. Body
Creating a Nonanxious Presence (R – RE – CR)
Titration Part I: Trigger List Using Braking and Acceleration (R – RE – CR)
Progressive Relaxation (R)
Autogenics (R – CR)
Diaphragmatic Breathing (R)
3-6 Breathing (R)
5-4-3-2-1 Sensory Grounding and Containment (R)
Postural Grounding (R)
Anchoring Part I: Collapsing Anchors (R)

3. Cognition
Anchoring Part II: Safety (R)
Safe-Place Visualization (R)
Positive Self-Talk and Thought Replacement/Transformation (CR)
Flashback Journal (R – RE)
Thought-Stopping (R – RE – CR)
Buddha's Trick (R – CR)

4. Behavior
Rituals (R – CR)
Contract for Safety and Self-Care (R – CR)
Safety Net Plan (R – CR)
Timed and Metered Expression Strategies (R – RE)

5. Emotion/Relation
Transitional Objects (R)
Support Systems (R – CR)
Drawing Icon and Envelope (Emotional Containment) (R – RE – CR)
Internal Vault (Emotional Containment) (R – RE – CR)
Positive Hope Box (R – RE – CR)

The effects of trauma reverberate through time and across a wide spectrum of life activities. Depending on the circumstances, these effects result in debilitating behaviors meant to alleviate anxiety that are often less than healthy and less than useful to that purpose. In other words, clients self-soothe in less-than-healthy ways. They may withdraw from life, use alcohol or drugs, or develop personality habits that are self-defeating. They may actually continue to place themselves in situations that are chaotic and anxiety provoking because they lack the skills and emotional stability to make better choices. They may show up on the doorstep of a therapist with every diagnosis in the Diagnostic and Statistical Manual of Mental Disorders (DSM) other than PTSD. In fact, many experienced therapists believe that almost all the symptoms they see in their practice are related to trauma in one way or another. It is important to understand that to accomplish the task of trauma symptom reduction the client must be able to create a state of relaxation. When their life is in chaos or they continue to self-soothe in less-than-useful ways, creating this state is next to impossible. Section 2 defines safety and provides techniques by which the practitioner can assist their clients in creating the environment of safety necessary for trauma work. There are techniques that address the elements of Body, Cognition, Behavior, and Emotions/Relationships essential to recovery.

1. What Is Safety?

In 1996, while completing a fellowship in psychotraumatology at West Virginia University in Morgantown, WV, Eric Gentry wrote an article on developing and maintaining safety with trauma survivors that was later published as a chapter in *Death and Trauma* (Figley, Bride, & Mazza, 1997). In this chapter, which provides a protocol for assessing and developing stabilization, Gentry attempts to define and "operationalize" the concept of safety into three levels relative to the treatment of trauma survivors. These three levels of safety are

- resolution of impending environmental (ambient, interpersonal, and intrapersonal) physical danger, including
  - removal from "war zone" (e.g., domestic violence, combat, abuse);
  - behavioral interventions to provide maximum safety;
  - addressing and resolving self-harm;
- amelioration of self-destructive thoughts and behaviors (e.g., suicidal/homicidal ideation/behavior, eating disorders, persecutory alters/ego-states, addictions, trauma-bonding, risk-taking behaviors, isolation);
- restructuring victim mythology into a proactive survivor identity by development and habituation of life-affirming self-care skills (e.g., daily routines, relaxation skills, grounding/containment skills, assertiveness, secure provision of basic needs, self-parenting).

One of the most difficult questions that a clinician must answer is: *What is the adequate level of safety/stability necessary to transition to Phase II (Trauma Memory Processing) of treatment?* We are taught from the first days of our clinical training to "above all do no harm" (*primum non nocere*), which makes it logical to assume that the more safety and stability that we, as clinicians, can affect in the lives of our clients, the better for their treatment – right?

The answer to this question can be a double-edged sword. For example, Gentry states that early in his career as a trauma therapist he spent many therapy hours working with clients to establish safety and stability. However, upon closer inspection, he saw this delay was his own anxiety about approaching the traumatic material that actually "escalated the crises of my clients." The safety issue was as much about his own emotional safety as that of his clients. So, how safe do you have to be and how do you get there? There are no hard-and-fast criteria for safety, but we will discuss various techniques to help establish safety and stabilization and discuss reference points that can be useful to help you decide.

It is a commonly held hypothesis among trauma therapists that the most important ingredient to effective establishment of stabilization and even treatment outcomes is the warm confidence of the clinician. A nonanxious presence, along with an unwavering optimism for the client's prognosis, is probably the most powerful intervention that you can provide toward the development of stabilization for your clients. However, you will find that destabilization and lack of safety is often precipitated by client behaviors and thoughts in response to the bombardment of intrusive symptoms (e.g., nightmares, flashbacks, psychological and physiological reactivity). A protracted period of attempting to overdevelop safety for these clients is not helpful. An approach is needed that develops the minimum ("good enough") level of safety and stabilization and then addresses and resolves the intrusive symptoms by enabling a narrative of the traumatic experience. This is often counterintuitive and almost always initially anxiety-producing for the clinician. However, the client will be much better equipped to change their self-destructive patterns (e.g., addictions, eating disorders, abusive relationships) with the intrusive symptoms resolved because they will have much more of their faculties available for intervention on their own behalf.

Minimum Criterion Required for Transition to Phase II Treatment

Again, what is the minimal standard of safety necessary to begin Phase II of treatment? While this question has not been addressed in the literature, much less resolved, we will propose the following criteria:

1. Resolution of impending environmental and physical danger (i.e., ambient, interpersonal, and intrapersonal). Level One of Safety, as previously discussed, must be achieved. Traumatic memories will not resolve if the client is in *active* danger and the clinician must use cognitive and especially behavioral treatments to assist the client in removing themselves from harm's way (see "Am Safe vs. Feel Safe" discussion below).

2. Ability to distinguish between "Am Safe" and "Feel Safe." Many trauma survivors feel as if danger lurks around every corner, at all times. In fact, the symptom cluster of "arousal" is mostly about this phenomenon. It is important for the clinician to confront this distortion and help the client to distinguish, objectively, between "outside danger" and "inside danger." Outside danger, or a "real" environmental threat, must be met with behavioral interventions designed to help the survivor remove or protect themselves from this danger. Inside danger, or the fear resultant from intrusive symptoms of past traumatic experiences, must be met with interventions designed to lower arousal and develop awareness and insight into the source (memory) of the fear (see Figure 4).

3. Development of a battery of self-soothing, grounding, containment, and expression strategies and *the ability to utilize them for self-rescue from intrusions.* These techniques should be taught during the early sessions prior to beginning Phase II of treatment. At a minimum, clients should be taught the following skills:
- 3-2-1 sensory grounding technique;
- visualization of a "safe place";
- progressive relaxation (and/or other anxiety-reduction skills);
- development of self-soothing discipline (e.g., working out, music, art, gardening, etc.);
- containment strategy(ies);
- expression strategy(ies).

These skills are explained in detail throughout this book.

4. Ability to practice-demonstrate self-rescue. It is useful to ask the client to begin to narrate their traumatic experience(s) and when they begin to experience intensifying affect, the clinician should challenge them to implement the skills above to demonstrate the ability to self-rescue from a full-blown flashback. This successful experience can then be utilized later in treatment to empower the client to extricate themself from overwhelming traumatic memories. It is also a testament to the client now being empowered with *choice* to continue treatment and confront trauma memories. The metaphor of teaching a novice sailor the procedures of sailing

Inside Danger	Outside Danger
Perceived Fear, No Present Danger CAN BEGIN TRAUMA WORK Anxiety Reduction Cognitive Restructuring Self-Soothing	Real Present Danger – DO NOT BEGIN TRAUMA WORK Behavioral Intervention Resolve Threat

Figure 4. Dealing with inside and outside danger.

mechanics prior to casting off so that they can assist with the management of the boat, instead of becoming a liability during rough seas, is a useful tool for explaining this important skill.

5. Positive prognosis and contract with client to address traumatic material. The final important ingredient of the Safety phase of treatment is negotiating the contract with the client to move forward to Phase II (Trauma Memory Processing). Remember from previous work the importance of mutual goals in the creation and maintenance of the therapeutic alliance. It is important for the clinician to harness the power of the client's willful intention to resolve the trauma memories before moving forward. An acknowledgment of the client's successful completion of the Safety phase of treatment, coupled with an empowering statement of positive prognosis, will most likely be helpful here (e.g., "I have watched you develop some very good skills to keep yourself safe and stable in the face of these horrible memories. Judging from how well you have done this, I expect the same kind of success as we begin to work toward resolving these traumatic memories. What do you need before we begin to resolve these memories?").

It is not necessary that the client meet all the objective criteria before moving to Phase II; however, the clinician should be able to interpret any shortcomings to ensure that there is no danger in moving ahead with treatment. "Red flags" or concerns about dissociative symptoms or potential regression should alert the clinician that movement forward might be premature. Warning signs may indicate that (a) the client needs more work toward the development of stabilization skills and/or (b) the client is experiencing a dissociative regression.

What follows are a variety of techniques useful for self-soothing, grounding, containment, and self-rescue. These are not the only techniques available, merely examples. Notice that they either subtly begin to incorporate the principle of reciprocal inhibition (relaxation and exposure), address the narrative of what occurs cognitively, or both.

For up-to-date information on training in the assessment of dissociation, regression, and chronic complex posttraumatic stress, please refer to the Traumatology Institute Training Curriculum – training programs available both online and face-to-face through http://www.psychink.com and http://www.ticlearn.com. The Traumatology Institute course TI-202 offers a systematic assessment method for aiding clinicians in determining readiness for trauma care.

2. Body

Traumatic events trigger a subsystem of the autonomic nervous system (ANS) called the *sympathetic nervous system* (SNS). This is a survival system that releases chemicals into the body and prepares it to fight, flee, or freeze. Although this is a normal sequence, it is an unpleasant experience characterized by fear, anxiety, and very high arousal. Remembering traumatic events can also trigger this cascade of chemicals, creating the same experience. Left unmanaged, this survival/fear response is counterproductive to the therapeutic process. There are a variety of ways to manage this sequence. This section provides body-based techniques that are useful in the management of the fear response.

Creating a Nonanxious Presence (R – RE – CR)

Time required: A few seconds, but repeated often until well learned.
Materials required: Yourself.

This technique is adapted from *A Language of the Heart: Therapy Stories that Heal*, by D. Franklin Schultz, PhD. It is designed to help create and maintain a nonanxious presence and is one of the easiest ways to manage stress. It uses the body itself to turn off the fear response by intentionally stimulating the *parasympathetic* nervous system (PNS). It is an intervention

Section 2: Safety and Stabilization

Indications for use: Use when the primary need is to manage the fear response. This is a self-soothing skill that can be utilized as required throughout the remainder of these techniques.
Counterindications: None.

that, once learned, can be used throughout the recovery process. It is a powerful and effective way for both the client *and* the therapist to manage immediate emotional overwhelm such as fear, anger, and sadness. It combines both physiological and cognitive resources to turn off the survival response.

The first part is primarily psychoeducational for the client. When they understand the sequence of events in their brain related to the survival response, they are better able to normalize the process. In other words, they realize they are not broken when this response occurs – they are normal. And they understand there is a normal intervention they can use to manage it. However, it is a technique that needs to be practiced daily until it becomes almost second nature. Clients *and* therapists should practice it often, whether they think they need to or not. The more they practice it, the more profound the effect will be.

Delivery of Approach

1. What follows is a script for explaining to clients, in simple terms, the mechanism in the brain responsible for most of their difficulties. It contains a three-step exercise that only takes a few seconds to accomplish. For it to be effective, it is useful to practice the exercise often and before they might actually need to use it. A useful practice routine will be presented after the script.

Nonanxious Presence Script

Pre-script Psychoeducation

Our brain is layered, with different functions associated with each layer. The middle part of our brain is an old animal part that even primitive animals possess to some degree. This area is where all of our sensory information goes first. Everything we see, smell, taste, touch, and hear passes through the midbrain. This is where our emotions (sadness, fear, anger, etc.) are located. It is also where the survival routines (fight, flight, or freeze) are triggered.

Layered on top of the midbrain is the part most people imagine when they think of human brains – the part with squiggly lines running across it. This is called the *neocortex*. The neocortex contains functions that make us uniquely human. This is where the language areas are located, so it allows us to put words to our experiences. It is also where the logic areas are located, so it allows us to connect the dots, make sense of experiences, and attach meaning to events. In addition, it contains a function that allows us to manage our emotions.

Under normal circumstances, information comes into the midbrain where it is quickly evaluated to determine if we are in danger. If we are not in danger, the information is sent to the neocortex, where words are added to it, sense is made of it, and it is stored for future reference as a memory. However, if we perceive danger or we are being overwhelmed by strong emotions, the midbrain triggers survival routines and begins to prepare the body for fight, flight, or freeze. This preparation is accomplished by chemical messengers that flood through the body and prepare it to either run fast, fight hard, or submit by freezing to survive. You may be familiar with some of these chemicals: they are adrenaline, noradrenaline, aldosterone, and cortisol. This preparation for survival is responsible for the experience of the "adrenaline rush."

The following is a partial list of the things that happen in the body when these chemicals prepare it for survival:

1. The digestive process turns off. (There is no need to be wasting energy digesting food when you are running for your life.)
2. The immune system is depressed. (Again, immunity is a waste of energy if the goal is survival.)

3. Blood is pushed from the outer part of the body to the large muscle groups to provide them with energy (oxygen and food) to either fight, flee, or freeze. (To accomplish this, the heart rate increases and blood pressure increases.)
4. Sugar and cholesterol enter the blood to provide energy to the muscles.

If you think for a minute, you may find these reactions familiar. This is because they all happen to relate to the symptoms of long-term stress. What we call "stress" is really just the physiological experience of the survival sequence being triggered repeatedly. In other words, if the body drops into survival mode again and again, this sequence of events leads to the symptoms of long-term stress. For instance, when the digestive system is repeatedly compromised, symptoms such as ulcers, irritable bowel syndrome, gastritis, constipation, etc. occur. When the immune system is repeatedly compromised, we end up with infectious diseases, such as colds and flu. Even cancer and ulcers are now being associated with a compromised immune system. We end up with high blood pressure, high heart rate, and high cholesterol. More recent research even suggests that a form of diabetes may also be associated with the constant release of sugar from stress.

There is, however, one more very important event that occurs when we enter survival mode. Cortisol floods through the neocortex, essentially shutting down those functions that make us uniquely human. We lose the ability to think clearly. We lose the ability to find words to express ourselves precisely. Most important, we lose the ability to manage our emotions. You have probably seen people who become enraged, turn beet red, and yell an obscenity. This is the process that accounts for such things as "road rage." It occurs partly because their neocortex has begun to shut down and they do not have access to the words they need to actually articulate their inner experience or communicate what they want – n or do they have access to the logic areas or the ability to manage their emotions. When we are in survival mode, it is extremely difficult to actually think about what is going on and choose our next response, instead of just making a knee-jerk reaction. In other words, when our neocortex is shut down, it is very difficult to be intentional.

It is a fact, however, that you cannot be stressed and relaxed at the same time. When you are in danger mode, the SNS is activated. This subsystem is responsible for sending out the chemical messengers, increasing your heart rate and blood pressure, tensing your muscles, making your breathing shallower, and shutting down your digestive and immune systems. Conversely, the PNS does everything in reverse of the SNS. The PNS turns off the survival response, thereby lowering your heart rate and blood pressure, etc. Intentionally activating the PNS essentially shuts down the SNS, c onfirming that you cannot, in fact, be stressed and relaxed at the same time.

Script

The following is a three-step exercise designed to help you activate your PNS. The first step will probably sound familiar because we are told to do it over and over by others when we seem upset. However, we are rarely taught steps 2 and 3, which actually make step 1 work.

Step 1
To begin, take a slow deep breath. What part of you moved when you took it? If you said your chest, you are probably breathing from the top of your lungs. When you take a deep breath, your diaphragm should drop down and push your belly out of the way. This is the normal way to breathe. If you watch a baby breathe – before it has been told to hold in that belly – you will notice the belly rise and fall. When you breathe from the top of your lungs, you only move a small percentage of the air from your lungs. When you breathe into your belly, you move a vastly higher percentage of the air a nd, by so doing, you put more oxygen into your blood stream. The first step of the exercise is to take a single, slow, deep belly breath.

Now, before you go to step 2, mentally go inside your body. This is a one-time internal check for tension. Start at your head and move all the way to your toes and back again. The object is to see where you are holding tension. Do not try and relax it right now, just take an inventory of where you hold it. Some people have tight shoulder or neck muscles. Some people hold tension in their chest, arms, or stomach. Some try and push their foot through the floor. Note how your body feels when you are paying attention to your tension.

Next, find the front part of your hipbones that jut out below your belly button. Then, notice where your buttock bones are located (this is the one you sit on). If you stood up, you could imagine lines that run down the front of your body from the level of your hipbones to the level of your buttock bones. Continue the lines back to your buttock bones, then up the back to the level of your hipbones and across again to the front where you started. You have just created an imaginary box that begins just below your belly button and extends down into your lower torso. Medical professionals would call this the *pelvic floor*. Martial artists, especially those who practice a martial art called Aikido, would call this the *one-point*. It is the balance and power point of the body.

Step 2
Now, take a deep belly breath. As you slowly exhale, intentionally relax this area called the one-point. That is, relax all the muscles that begin about two inches below the belly button. Now *really* relax it! Let the muscles in the front of your torso become soft enough to touch your backbone. What did you notice? If you have successfully relaxed the one-point, you should notice that your whole body immediately relaxes, including the parts where you have been holding tension.

Now do the exercise again, slowly. This time, pay close attention to what happens inside your head when you relax your one-point. Most people report what feels like a clear spot opening. Some report it feels like tension is being released from the sides out. You should also notice that you seem more clearheaded and better able to think. It is a very simple exercise: take one deep breath and (most important) relax your one-point – the belly muscles two inches below your belly button.

This is a very stable place to be. From this position of a relaxed one-point, you are able to experience powerful emotions such as sadness, fear, anxiety, and anger without having to "do" anything. You have the ability to feel your emotions and you can let them flow through you like water through a hose. In other words, you are in a state where you can decide (consciously intend) what you will do next.

Although it seems too simple, there are sound physiological reasons why this exercise works. Intentionally relaxing your body has one very important consequence: it stimulates the PNS, which turns off the SNS. Remember, you cannot be stressed and relaxed at the same time. When your body is relaxed, the midbrain is no longer delivering the message that you are in danger.

Did you know that zebras do not get ulcers?[1] Ulcers are frequently one of the symptoms humans experience from unrelenting stress. They result from a physical reaction caused by the midbrain constantly telling the body it is in danger and to prepare to survive. One of the ways it prepares the body for survival is by chemically turning off the digestive process because there is no need to be wasting energy digesting food when you are running for your life. When this occurs repeatedly, symptoms such as ulcers occur (also irritable bowel syndrome, gastritis, constipation, etc.). You would think that being chased across the Savannah by a large lion would create enough stress to cause an ulcer. But, as it turns out, zebras do not get ulcers (yes, the study has been conducted!). Here is why: after zebras are finished

---
[1] See Sapolsky (2004).

being chased by the lion, they eat their lunch! In other words: no lion, no stress. They live in the here and now; after the lion is gone, their midbrains are no longer preparing their body to survive.

Humans, on the other hand, remember the lion that chased them yesterday and fantasize about the lion that will chase them tomorrow. In fact, many people go looking for lions to worry about because feeling like they are in danger is what they consider normal. There is never a time when their midbrain is not telling them they are in danger, and it is the physical reaction to constantly being in "danger" that results in symptoms like ulcers. Understanding this, you can now add step 3.

Step 3
Now that you have taken a deep breath and relaxed your belly muscles, take a moment to notice what happens inside your head and ask yourself, "Am I safe?" Right here, right now, right this second, are you safe? No lions, no stress...

This exercise is most effective when practiced often and before it is needed. The following routine has been found useful in acquiring the skill of being nonanxious. Take a business card and write on the back of it "relax your belly." Place the card where you are likely to see it throughout the day as often as 10 or 15 times (on a computer screen, in a pocket, next to your credit card). Make the agreement with yourself that every time you see the card, think of the card, or touch the card, you will do the exercise. This means you will take a moment to take a slow deep breath, let it out slowly as you relax your belly, notice what happens inside your head and ask, "am I safe?"

Clients are likely to notice the following sequence of events. The first couple of days they will notice that each time they do the exercise they will find themselves relaxing more and more. This is because they are literally training their body to relax on command, which it is not used to doing. After doing the exercise 10 or 15 times a day for a week or more, they will also begin to notice something else: the body does not like being tense. When it finds a way to relax itself it will begin doing so spontaneously. They will find themselves spontaneously taking a deep breath and relaxing. And when this happens, many will notice something else. When they are experiencing a strong emotion (fear, anger, sadness) and they do the exercise, an interesting thing happens: the emotion does not disappear. However, they suddenly will not have to *do* anything about it. They will be able to watch it flow through them like water flows through a hose and they will not have to *do* anything. The neocortex will be functioning and the feeling of overwhelm will subside. This is a powerful and healing place from which to continue recovery.

Titration Part I: Trigger List Using Braking and Acceleration (R – RE – CR)

Time required: One or more sessions depending on the extensiveness of the trauma.
Materials required: Pencil and paper (or the following chart).
Indications for use: Use when the primary need is to enhance physical, cognitive, and emotional coping skills in the Safety and Stabilization stage of trauma recovery. The client

In her excellent book, *The Body Remembers*, Rothschild (2000) encourages clinicians to teach clients how to apply the "brakes" when beginning trauma therapy. She uses the analogy of teaching a new driver to be really comfortable with the braking system in a car before accelerating. In the same manner, she finds methods for teaching clients how to "brake" before becoming deeply involved in trauma work. In this way, the client moderates the trauma work. A client can begin their work beyond fear after they have learned that they need not be stuck in fear forever. After an individual learns that they can touch just the surface of their experience and then return to a safe or neutral ground, it is empowering and affords them the knowledge that they can master their own discomfort.

| Section 2: Safety and Stabilization | 35 |

will have been taught or can demonstrate self-soothing skills that can be utilized as required throughout the development of the Trigger List in this exercise. **Counterindications:** If client is clearly unstable, labile, actively dissociating, or dissociates during exercise.

There are many ways to apply the brakes as a way of moderating the release process involved in trauma therapy. In this section, we will review many braking methods, including: Deep Beathing, Muscle Relaxation, Comfort in One Part, Safe-Place Imaging, Anchoring, Transitional Objects/Memories/Figures, etc. The idea is to be aware of many approaches because something may work for one person but not another. Layering (Baranowsky, 1997), which is taught in the next section, is a Braking and Accelerating exercise that has been found to be very useful in a clinical setting as well as on a trauma/disaster site. The key with this approach is to start and stop trauma review so processing is not overly explosive or extreme for the individual.

Delivery of Approach

Here is an example of a titration of significant traumatic events that occur over a lifetime. In this example, the client reviews their life chronologically, identifying significant disturbing life experiences with short, simple descriptions in order from birth to the present.

1. **Time-Out:** Discuss time-out or stop signs with your client. This can simply be a raised hand (stop sign/time-out) to let you know a break is needed. This will indicate it is time for a temporary change of subject or pause in discussion to reclaim one's comfort.
2. **Trigger List:** Work with your client to develop a Trigger List of disturbing life experiences that continue to feel unresolved, upsetting, and traumatic.
3. **Break-Down:** The Trigger List is to be broken down into early childhood, middle childhood to adolescence, young adulthood, and adulthood to the present (complete sections as required by the client's age and experiences).
4. **Using Brakes:** After you have begun this list, ensure that you remind the client to stop and apply the brakes whenever things feel overwhelming. This "putting on the brakes" will give the client the opportunity to practice some self-soothing techniques and demonstrate for themselves, during the session, their ability to manage symptoms before they become overwhelming.
5. **Create Guardrails:** Ensure that the client provides one-sentence, simple descriptions (maximum 10 words) that are just enough to recall the memory without going into great detail – that will come later (e.g., I was 12 years old, in front of my family home. It was the day I walked across the street and was struck by a motorist). The first few words just give the time frame and context. It is the words that follow that identify the traumatic memory and they are not to exceed 7–10 words.
6. **SUDs Rating:** After the list is complete, read all the memories back to the client, giving the client a chance to reflect on them and rate them based on the Subjective Units of Distress scale (SUDs). This is a 1-to-10 scale where 1 represents a calm relaxed state, 5 represents discomfort but within a manageable range, and 10 is the worst feelings of distress the person can recall. Explain the SUDs scale so they can give you the number that best reflects their feelings of distress now, in this moment, when they think of that difficult moment from the past. The list is to be completed based on how the individual feels as they look back on the event now.
7. **Add till Complete:** Allow the individual to add as many memories as they wish to each section until they feel it is complete.
8. **Identify Themes:** After the trigger list has been built, reflect again on all of the items on the list to identify any "guiding principles" or core beliefs that stand out or appear in various forms through significant life experiences. These may take the form of negative beliefs (e.g., I am not loveable; everyone lets me down; life is dangerous). These are the operating principles upon which a person is building their beliefs about the world around them and have a fundamental impact on how they walk on this earth.

Consider the following abbreviated trigger-list example:

USING THE TOOLS: EXAMPLE
Trigger-List Exercise (Multiple Events)

Life stage	Trigger List	SUDs
Early childhood*		
1. Age 10	Teased in school yard because of weight	8
2. Age 12	Three boys corner me and molest me on way home from school	10
3. Age 12	Parents do not want to talk about what happened after police leave the house	10
4. Age 27	Weight-loss doctor shames me for being unable to stay on a diet	7

After reviewing all the items above and rating the memories the client is asked to reflect on the Themes. The list following below are the Themes identified by the client based on the Trigger List developed and rated above:

- I am not acceptable as I am.
- I am unlovable.
- No one will accept me once they know me.
- People are cruel.

Now it is possible to work with both the memories and the core beliefs that have been established as a result of these pivotal life experiences.

Note: This approach is similar to the Time-Line approach in the Trauma Memory Processing section, but is strictly used to capture the memory rather than to process at this stage.

USING THE TOOLS
Trigger-List Exercise (Multiple Events)

Life stage	Trigger List	SUDs
Early childhood*		
1.		
2.		
3.		
Middle childhood to adolescence*		
1.		
2.		
3.		
Young adulthood*		
1.		
2.		
3.		
Adulthood to present day*		
1.		
2.		
3.		

List of themes (or core beliefs):

1. _____

2. _____

3. _____

* Use additional pages if necessary

Note: This page may be reproduced by the purchaser for clinical use.

From: Anna B. Baranowsky, J. Eric Gentry, & D. Franklin Schultz, *Trauma Practice: Tools for Stabilization and Recovery.* © 2011 Hogrefe Publishing

USING THE TOOLS
Trigger-List Exercise (One Event – Multiple Hot Points)

Use this Trigger List in a graphical manner when there is one event that occurred over a long period of time with multiple "hot points" or disturbing moments related to the same event.

Example:

	1	2	3	4	5	6	7	8	9	10

Start

Driving in a snow storm — 4

Car cuts me off and I skid but I'm okay — 7

Snow starts to reduce — 4

Hit black ice and lose control of car — 9

Car flips in ditch — 10

I'm alive, not badly injured — 7

Ambulance & police arrive — 4

At hospital, informed of internal injuries — 9

Family arrives for support — 4

Doctors give good news about surgery — 4

Note: This page may be reproduced by the purchaser for clinical use.

From: Anna B. Baranowsky, J. Eric Gentry, & D. Franklin Schultz, *Trauma Practice: Tools for Stabilization and Recovery.* © 2011 Hogrefe Publishing

Progressive Relaxation (R)

Time required: 5–30 minutes, depending on script.
Materials required: None.
Indications for use: Use when the primary need is to enhance physical coping skills in the Safety and Stabilization stage of trauma recovery. Our body's nervous system is the key to healing from trauma. When we teach body calmness, we teach disengagement from hyperalert and overanxious responses of a stressed system. This is a step toward body retraining.
Counterindications: Actively dissociating or dissociates during exercise.

Delivery of Approach

Ehrenreich (1999) provides a simple script for Progressive Relaxation that can be expanded with minimal effort. Begin this exercise by instructing the individual to focus on lengthening and deepening the breath. Focus on the inhalation and exhalation making the breath smooth and deep.

Now tighten both fists, and tighten your forearms and biceps ... Hold the tension for five or six seconds ... Now relax the muscles. When you relax the tension, do it suddenly, as if you are turning off a light ... Concentrate on the feelings of relaxation in your arms for 15 or 20 seconds ... Now tense the muscles of your face and tense your jaw ... Hold it for five or six seconds ... now relax and concentrate on the relaxation for 15 or 20 seconds ... Now arch your back and press out your stomach as you take a deep breath ... Hold it ... and relax ... Now tense your thighs and calves and buttocks ... Hold ... and now relax. Concentrate on the feelings of relaxation throughout your body, breathing slowly and deeply (Ehrenreich, 1999, Appendix B).

From the brief description above, the clinician can encourage tightness and relaxation throughout the body, from top to bottom or in any order they prefer. The body is progressively released and relaxed throughout.

Autogenics (R – CR)

Time required: 10–20 minutes, depending on script.
Materials required: Script.
Indications for use: Use when the primary need is to enhance physical coping skills in the Safety and Stabilization stage of trauma recovery.
Counterindications: Actively dissociating or dissociates during exercise.

Autogenics is a slightly different form of self-induced relaxation than Progressive Relaxation. Rather than using the muscles to tighten and then release, Autogenics focuses on using one's own self-talk related to the body to produce a very deep sense of relaxation. A favorite script for Autogenic Relaxation comes from *Mastering Chronic Pain* (Jamison, 1996). This book, though written for a different audience, provides an excellent deep-relaxation script.

Autogenics is not hypnosis per se because, as the name itself suggests, (auto)effects are produced by the individual. In fact, the script offers an ideal process for learning to use *internal* dialogue to calm and soothe the internal world. The individual is in control of the process the entire time. However, Autogenics *is* a very powerful technique that is capable of self-inducing a dreamlike, calm state in the individual. As you read the script to the client, take your time to inhale fully and read a line on the exhalation. This breathing-paced reading aids the clinician in sending a relaxing message to the client, further enhancing their experience. It also allows the client time to silently repeat the statement back to themselves while you inhale slowly. This technique would be counterindicated for clients who are already dissociative or for those you suspect are dissociative. In cases where the clinician or counselor does not have sufficient training with Dissociative Disorders, it is best to make the decision to teach the use of Autogenics with caution.

Delivery of Approach

It is helpful to walk the client through the process the first time when using a script that you can later hand to them for their own use. Encourage the client to find a relaxing place and position before beginning the relaxation exercise. Although it is useful to have one's eyes closed to enhance relaxation, it is not necessary. Begin to focus on the breath. Start to soften, lengthen, and deepen the breath. Let it become the focus of attention. Recognize that relaxation is a process and occurs over time as one begins to let go of tension and tightness.

When finished with the script, encourage the client to bring their attention back into the room in which they are relaxing. Suggest that they can bring feelings of relaxation into their regular day simply by focusing in the same manner as they have during this exercise. Close by asking the person you are working with to slowly bring their attention fully back, taking their time. It is important to inform your client that, when using the technique, they will be very relaxed. They should spend an appropriate amount of time grounding themselves to the here-and-now before attempting to stand or perform complicated tasks such as driving.

USING THE TOOLS
Autogenic Relaxation

The script for autogenic relaxation below is reproduced with the author's permission from *Mastering Chronic Pain: A Professional's Guide to Behavioral Treatment* (pp. 73–74), by R. N. Jamison, 1996. He begins with: "Now slowly, in your mind, repeat to yourself each of the phrases I say to you. Focus on each phrase as you repeat it to yourself".

I am beginning to feel calm and quiet.
I am beginning to feel quite relaxed.
My right foot feels heavy and relaxed.
My left foot feels heavy and relaxed.
My ankles, knees, and hips feel heavy, relaxed, and comfortable.
My stomach, chest, and back feel heavy and relaxed.
My neck, jaw, and forehead feel completely relaxed.
All of my muscles feel comfortable and smooth.
My right arm feels heavy and relaxed.
My left arm feels heavy and relaxed.
My right hand feels heavy and relaxed.
My left hand feels heavy and relaxed.
Both my hands feel heavy and relaxed.
My breathing is slow and regular.
I feel very quiet.
My whole body is relaxed and comfortable.
My heartbeat is calm and regular.
I can feel warmth going down into my right hand.
It is warm and relaxed.
My hands are warm and heavy.
It would be very difficult to raise my hands at this moment.
I feel very heavy.
My breathing is slow and deep.
My breathing is getting deeper and deeper.
I am feeling calm.
My whole body is heavy, warm, and relaxed.
My whole body feels very quiet and comfortable.
My mind is still, calm, and cool.
My body is warm and relaxed.
My breathing is deeper and deeper.
I feel secure and still.
I am completely at ease.
I feel an inner peace.
I am breathing more and more deeply.

Note: This page may be reproduced by the purchaser for clinical use.

From: Anna B. Baranowsky, J. Eric Gentry, & D. Franklin Schultz, *Trauma Practice: Tools for Stabilization and Recovery.* © 2011 Hogrefe Publishing

Diaphragmatic Breathing (R)

Time required: 5 minutes.
Materials required: None.
Indications for use: Use when the primary need is to enhance physical coping skills in the Safety and Stabilization stage of trauma recovery.
Counterindications: Any respiratory complications.

If we watch an infant sleep, we will see the rhythmical movement of deep belly breathing. This is the ideal breathing for relaxation and the nourishing of the body with the breath.

When we feel upset or anxious about something, our breathing is often the first thing to change. It is likely to become shallow, rapid, and jagged or raspy. If, on the other hand, we were to practice intentional Diaphragmatic Breathing, we would be more able to consciously regulate our breathing when we become upset.

Delivery of Approach

Find a comfortable, unrestricting position in which to sit or lie. Place your hands on your belly as a guide to the breath. Begin to consciously slow and smooth out the breath. Notice the rhythm of the breath through the inhalation and exhalation. Is it smooth, deep, and full, or jagged, shallow, and slight? Now focus on bringing a deeper breath into the belly. Let a full breath be released upon exhalation. Inhale fully, not holding the breath at any time. On the exhalation release completely and pause, counting to three after the exhalation is complete. Then inhale slowly, fully, and deeply. Continue to focus in this manner on the breath.

Gentry suggests placing one's clasped hands behind the neck. This opens the chest through the lifting and spreading of the elbows. As this occurs, breath moves much more freely, deep into the belly. This procedure is an excellent alternative (to hands on the belly) for those just learning deep breathing exercises.

At first, the individual is taught to deep-breathe in sets of five. Then this is increased to 10 inhalations and exhalations. Finally, an instruction is given to practice two times each day for 5 minutes per day. In this way, the individual is learning to relax through deep breathing.

3-6 Breathing (R)

Time required: 20 minutes.
Materials required: This can be used in conjunction with a biofeedback system like the EmWave® Coherence System that is available through http://www.heartmath.com. This system allows the client to receive immediate feedback both before and after breath training so they can monitor their progress and see improvement as a result of training. Although biofeedback is an excellent resource, it is possible to effectively teach 3-6 Breathing without any equipment.
Indications for use: Use when the primary need is to enhance physical coping skills in the Safety and Stabilization stage of trauma recovery.
Counterindications: Any respiratory complications.

Delivery of Approach

At the start of this exercise it is best to focus all your attention internally and, if possible, it is preferable to begin with your eyes closed. When you are focusing on your breath, sit or lie in a relaxed position where you are comfortable and will not be disrupted. Please note that a full breath is considered an inhalation and an exhalation.

USING THE TOOLS
3-6 Breathing

1. *Noticing:* Instruct your client to "just notice the pace, depth, and movement of the breath as you take three inhalations and exhalations (three breaths). Notice if the breath is deep, shallow, smooth, or rough and how it feels moving in and out of the body." After three breaths, ask your client to report on the experience of the breath.

   Capture Client Response

   _____

   _____

2. *Deepening:* Instruct your client to "just notice by focusing that you can make the breath deeper, smoother, and slower. Take three breaths again, being careful not to hold your breath at any time. When you get to the edge of a full inhalation, begin to exhale without straining the body at any time. Bring the breath deep into the belly on the inhalation and release the breath completely on the exhalation, letting the body rest for a beat at the end of the exhalation before inhaling again. At the end of the third exhalation, let me know when you are done and what it feels like to deepen, slow, and smooth out the breath."

   Capture Client Response

   _____

   _____

3. *Sipping:* Now prepare your client to work with a sipping breath by instructing them to "imagine that there is a straw in your mouth and you are inhaling through that straw very slowly and smoothly. N – otice that you can bring the breath deep into your belly. At the edge of the inhalation, begin to exhale through the nose. Do not hold or force the breath. Do this three times and tell me when you are done and what this felt like."

   Capture Client Response

   _____

   _____

4. *Counting:* Now add another instruction (demonstrate for your client the count of three on the inhalation and six on the exhalation, – counting with your fingers so that the exhalation is twice as long as the exhalation; y – ou will have to practice this rhythm until it is comfortable for you and easy to demonstrate). Now "following my example, begin to inhale slowly, fully, and deeply into the belly to the count of three and release slowly and completely to the count of six (counting in your own mind). Staying focused on the slow, full rhythm of inhalation and exhalation, do this five times and tell me when you are done."

   Capture Client Response

   _____

   _____

5. *Biofeedback using EmWave®:* If you are using the EmWave® system or any other biofeedback system, begin this session by taking a silent 3-minute baseline of performance. After breath training, take another 3-minute reading of the performance to compare and contrast for the client. It is often amazing the progress that is achieved and can be demonstrated for the client within a short time period using this pattern of breath training.

Note: This page may be reproduced by the purchaser for clinical use.

From: Anna B. Baranowsky, J. Eric Gentry, & D. Franklin Schultz, *Trauma Practice: Tools for Stabilization and Recovery.* © 2011 Hogrefe Publishing

5-4-3-2-1 Sensory Grounding and Containment (R)

Time required: 7 minutes.
Materials required: None.
Indications for use: Use when the primary need is to enhance physical and emotional coping skills in the Safety and Stabilization stage of trauma recovery.
Counterindications: None.

This technique assists the trauma survivor in developing the capacity to "self-rescue" from the obsessive, hypnotic, and numinous power of traumatic intrusions and flashbacks. It is based on the assumption that if the survivor is able to break their absorbed internal attention to the traumatic images, thoughts, and feelings by instead focusing on and connecting with their current external surroundings through their senses (here and now), the accompanying fight-or-flight arousal will diminish. This technique will assist the survivor in understanding that they are perfectly safe in their present context and in understanding the value of using their sensory skills (sight, touch, smell, hearing, and taste) to "ground" them to this safety in the present empirical reality.

Delivery of Approach

1. Begin by asking the client to tell part of their trauma narrative and allow them to begin to experience some affect (e.g., reddening of eyes, psychomotor agitation, constricted posture).
2. When they have begun to experience some affect (~ 5 on a SUDs scale), ask them "would you like some help out of those uncomfortable images, thoughts, and feelings?"
3. If they answer yes, ask them to describe, out loud, five objects that they can see in the room. Make certain that these are physical and not imagined objects.
4. Ask them to identify, out loud, five "real world" sounds that they can currently hear while sitting in the room (the sound can be beyond the room, just make certain that they are empirical and not from the traumatic material).
5. Hand them any item (a pen, notebook, Kleenex), and ask them to thoroughly feel it and to describe, out loud, the texture of this object. Repeat this with four additional objects.
6. Return to objects that they can see and ask them to now identify four objects that they can see. Do the same with things that they can hear and feel (instead of handing items to the client, ask them to reach out, touch, and describe the texture of two objects). Repeat this until you reach one object each for sight, sound, and texture.
7. When completed, ask the client, "What happened with the traumatic material?" Most of the time your client will describe a significant lessening of negative feelings, thoughts, and images associated with the traumatic material.

Note: For many survivors, this technique will mark the first time that they have been able to rescue themselves from a flashback or traumatic material. It is often an experience of tremendous empowerment because it can represent the *"beginning of the end of victimization"* for the survivor. The clinician may want to allow ample opportunity to explore this process and utilize the "teachable moment" inherent in this process.

Postural Grounding (R)

Time required: 5 minutes.
Materials required: None.
Indications for use: Use when the primary need is to enhance physical coping skills in the Safety and Stabilization stage of trauma recovery.
Counterindications: Severe physical injury, disability, or impairment.

Postural Grounding is a technique drawn from practice with clients who have dissociative symptoms. As a trauma survivor begins to experience the images and feelings associated with a flashback, they can often be observed to migrate into a constricted and fetal posture of protection. In addition, the clinician can usually notice psychomotor agitation in the form of shaking legs, tremors, either fixated or scanning eyes, and shallow breathing.

Delivery of Approach

When the client begins exhibiting these signs of reexperiencing and arousal, ask them "Would you like some help in getting out of there [those images and feelings]?" If the client says yes, follow the script below to help them develop the capacity for self-rescue from flashbacks.

1. While the client is exhibiting the constricted and fetal posture or some other physical posture indicates a fight, flight, or freeze response, ask them, "How vulnerable to do feel right now in that posture?" You will usually get an answer like "very."
2. Ask them to exaggerate this posture of constriction and protection (i.e., becoming more fetal) and then to take a moment to really experience and memorize the feelings currently in the muscles of their body.
3. Next, ask them to, "stand up, turn around, and then sit back down with an *adult* posture – one that feels in control." (It is helpful for the clinician to do this with the client as a demonstration.).
4. Ask them to exaggerate this posture of being in control and to really notice and memorize the feeling in the muscles of their body.
5. Ask them to articulate the difference between the two postures.
6. Ask them to shift several times between the two postures and to notice the different feelings, thoughts, and images associated with the two opposite postures.
7. Indicate to the client that they are now able to utilize this technique anytime that they feel overwhelmed by posttraumatic symptoms – especially in public places.
8. Discuss with the client opportunities where they will be able to practice this technique and make plans with them for its utility.

Anchoring Part I: Collapsing Anchors (R)

Time required: 10–20 minutes.
Materials required: None.
Indications for use: Use when the primary need is to enhance physical, cognitive, and emotional coping skills in the Safety and Stabilization stage of trauma recovery.
Counterindications: Actively dissociating or dissociates during exercise.

NLP Anchoring Script for Safety and Confidence
(Adapted from Bandler & Grinder, 1979; Reprint from Gentry & Baranowsky, 1998)

This exercise assists the individual to use the body (thumb, fingers, etc.) to "anchor" positive resource states. In doing so, the person learns to access these positive states more readily by capturing the memory in simple hand gestures. Other body parts can also be taught to be anchors for various resource states or memories.

Delivery of Approach

Relaxation induction. Find a comfortable spot where you can quietly begin to relax in the knowledge that you are in a safe place where you can release any of the tensions you hold. Allow your eyes to soften and the eyelids to rest lightly on the eyes. Begin to focus on the rhythm of your breath. Pay attention to how it flows into your body and then out again. Notice that with just a bit of effort you can lengthen the inhalation, making it smooth and soft. Imagine that it is a cool stream slowly filling the lower part of your belly – filling it completely. As the breath is released, allow any tensions to flow out with the exhalation. Inhale cool soothing breath, slowly filling up the belly; notice the belly rise. Exhale completely, releasing any tensions with the breath. Allow your eyes to close completely at this time if they are not already closed. Pause before the next inhalation, allowing even more breath to release and, along with it, tensions and toxins from the body. Recognize how the body begins to feel a greater sense of relaxation just by following the inhalations and exhalations. Notice how deepening the breath enhances feelings of well-being. Be aware that you can use this breath at any time in your day to enhance feelings of well-being, clarity, and focus. Notice that with each exhalation you feel a greater sense of inner peace and calmness. Remember that this is a tool you can use anywhere and any time in your regular day. Allow the inhalation and exhalation to become secondary – still smooth and deep but no longer the center of your attention.

Safety anchor. Now search your memory for a time when you felt great feelings of safety and reassurance. You may choose to use a comforting and safe place from real-life experience or one completely based on your imagination where you feel safe, comfortable, and relaxed. Recall all the contextual cues, such as sights, smells, sounds, air temperature, texture of objects, and anything else you are aware of. Identify the "exact moment" in this situation when you felt the greatest amount of safety. Become aware of the internal dialogue at that moment of safety. What was your mind saying during that time of great reassurance and security? What sensations did your body have when it felt this safety and joy and the freedom of relaxation? As this sensation reaches its height, squeeze together the thumb and forefinger on your dominant hand to anchor this experience of safety.

Competency or confidence anchor. Now allow your mind to recall a time in your past where you felt confident and competent. Memorize all the contextual clues such as sights, smells, sounds, temperature of the air, texture of objects, and any other contextual clues. Identify the "exact moment" in this situation when you felt the maximum amount of confidence and competence. Identify and experience what your mind was saying when you enjoyed these feelings of confidence and competence. What sensations were bodily felt when you experienced that great confidence and competence? What was it like to feel that potency? As this sensation of competence and confidence reaches its height, squeeze together the thumb and middle finger on your dominant hand to anchor this experience of competence and confidence.

Closure. Recognize that you can utilize these anchors at any time in your day when you feel stressed or upset. You can draw feelings of safety and confidence to enhance your access to personal resources and resiliency skills. Shortly, but not yet, you will be bringing your awareness back to this room with the knowledge that when you do you will feel fully refreshed and able to continue with the rest of your day – wiser, stronger, and more inwardly calm in the knowledge of your greater claim to inner resources. *As you make your way back to this room, you can begin to have feeling in your hands and feet ... arms and legs ... chest and stomach.* Lengthen and stretch through to your arms, hands, legs, and feet. You can begin to become more present behind your eyes. Take a deep breath and, when you are ready, open your eyes to normal waking consciousness.

3. Cognition

The brain and the mind are not the same thing, although they are intricately connected. Each affects the other in ways that are only partially understood. The physical brain can overwhelm us when it perceives danger, drops into survival mode, and makes rational thought (cognition) and behavior difficult. Conversely, our cognitive mind (the things we think, the way we interpret reality, and the way we talk to ourselves about it) can circumvent this process. When we have good control of our thinking process, we can avert that survival routine. The use of mental images and stories, the language we use in describing ourselves and the world to ourselves, and the meaning we attach to events all have the power to change the fear response. This section provides cognitive techniques for managing the fear response.

Anchoring Part II: Safety (R)

Time required: 10 minutes.
Materials required: None.
Indications for use: Use when the primary need is to enhance physical, cognitive, and emotional coping skills in the Safety and Stabilization stage of trauma recovery.
Counterindications: Actively dissociating or dissociates during exercise.

This exercise is an anchoring process that enables the individual to gain access to a safety state without the use of hypnosis-type exercises.

USING THE TOOLS
Anchoring Part II: Safety I

Safety Anchors

1. Instruct the client to identify a desired resource state (e.g., safety, courage, contentment).

   _____

   _____

2. Ask the client to identify a historical experience where the resource state was present.
   a. "Describe context" (i.e., at the cottage with the fireplace warming the room).

   _____

   _____

   b. Find the exact second that represents the resource state (i.e., place, time, objects, people present, etc.) Describe below:

   _____

   _____

   c. "Close eyes and reexperience" (10–15 seconds)

3. Make note of when the resource state was most intense. Describe below:

   _____

   _____

4. Behavioral
   a. "Close your eyes and imagine you are watching a videotape of this moment ..."
   b. "What would we see you doing ... specifically?"
   c. "What would be the look on your face?"
   d. Make note. Describe below:

   _____

   _____

5. Cognitive
   a. "Imagine that there is a tiny microphone that can listen to your thoughts at this moment ..."
   b. "What would we hear your mind say at the moment _____ (resource) is the strongest?"
   c. Make note. Describe below:

   _____

   _____

Note: These two pages may be reproduced by the purchaser for clinical use.

From: Anna B. Baranowsky, J. Eric Gentry, & D. Franklin Schultz, *Trauma Practice: Tools for Stabilization and Recovery.* © 2011 Hogrefe Publishing

6. Affective/Sensory
   a. "At the moment that _____ is the strongest …"
   b. "What do you feel in your body?"
   c. "What sensations do you experience?" Describe below:

   _____

   _____

7. Establish Anchor
   a. "Close your eyes and begin to experience _____ about 15 seconds before it reaches its 'peak' intensity."
   b. Narrate context.
   c. Narrate behavioral.
   d. Narrate cognitive.
   e. Narrate affect/sensory.
   f. "Allow this experience of _____ (resource state) to intensify even more … feel it expanding in your chest … in your mind …"

8. Trigger
   a. Now, squeeze together the thumb and forefinger of your dominant hand (5 seconds) … put all of the _____ into that squeeze."

9. Return to normal consciousness
   a. Test trigger ("How much of that feeling comes back when you squeeze your thumb and forefinger together now?") ____ %

Note: These two pages may be reproduced by the purchaser for clinical use.

From: Anna B. Baranowsky, J. Eric Gentry, & D. Franklin Schultz, *Trauma Practice: Tools for Stabilization and Recovery.* © 2011 Hogrefe Publishing

Safe-Place Visualization (R)

Time required: 5 – 30 minutes depending on script.
Materials required: Script.
Indications for use: Use when the primary need is to enhance cognitive and emotional coping skills in the Safety and Stabilization stage of trauma recovery.
Counterindications: Actively dissociating or dissociates during exercise.

The next exercise is not hypnosis, although it is a technique that utilizes some elements that are like "hypnotherapy." It is therefore limited for use by those who have had formal training and appropriate educational background to offer that type of work. This exercise is adapted from the *Treatment Manual for Accelerated Recovery from Compassion Fatigue* (Gentry & Baranowsky, 1998).

Delivery of Approach

Previsualization Information

Find a place and position where you can relax. This should be a place where you can be assured of minimal interruptions. Take the time to set the space for your maximum benefit. After you are satisfied with the environment and feel it will be one that is safe and relaxing, we will be ready to begin.

During this exercise you will have the opportunity to enjoy a sense of deep relaxation through a guided exercise. Through the exercise you will be instructed in the inner imagining of a Safe Place. This may be a place you have been to before or one entirely made up in your imagination.

Remember that this next exercise is a guided relaxation and imagery approach in which you remain in control while being deeply relaxed. You *can* stop at any time if you need to, *but* we recommend that you experience the entire exercise without interruptions to enjoy the greatest benefit and insight.

Focus on creating a sense of relaxation in the muscles in the back of your eyes and notice how this relaxation can spread. Now, as your eyelids softly rest over your eyes, notice how you are able to soften your facial muscles – first those that are closest to your eyes, but then more and more as you sense a smoothing, soothing, warming sensation spread across your face. Notice this warming, soothing sensation spread gently across your forehead ... across your eyes ... through your hairline. Notice as it warms and softens the lines of your face. Just notice and let the gentle warmth calm your face. This calming sensation moves down your face ... your nose ... lips ... chin ... until your whole face becomes a numb mass of relaxation. Even the mind takes on a soothing, mellow position ... until the mind feels very quiet. Listen to the sound of my voice and any other sounds without doing anything. Let these sounds be signals to let you know that you are safe, here in this room, allowing you to pay even closer attention to the *inside* world. Simply let the sounds assure you that you are in a safe place in this room. Feeling that safety, allow yourself to relax and slowly let the soothing warmth spread through to your neck muscles, helping you to release any tensions. The warmth now moves down through your arms all the way to your fingertips. As it does you can release tension in your upper body by imagining it spilling out through the tips of your fingers and into the ground below. Allow the warmth to spread through to your chest and fill up your lungs ... relaxing your muscles, relaxing your stomach, softening the muscles of the back and warming and releasing any tensions there. Continue to pay attention to my voice. Notice any points of tension and bring the soothing warmth to those points so they too can soften and relax. Bring the warmth through to your lower back, thigh, calves, feet, and toes. Become aware now that you can release even more tension from your lower body by imagining it spilling down all the way through to the tips of your toes and spilling out and into the ground. Just let your body relax as deeply as it wants, letting your conscious mind stray where it might ... and while your body relaxes it brings a feeling of calm detachment ... and a feeling that time doesn't matter, time is not important ... you feel calm and emotionally detached.

Safe-Place Imagery

Now allow your mind to find a relaxed and soothing space – a safe place. This is a place from the past that you have been to before or one from your imagination. Either way is okay, because it all belongs to you. Begin to develop a picture as a Polaroid film would develop. Watch as the safe place develops, exposing itself to you. Notice how the lights, colors, textures that surround you are now soothing to you. Notice what is above and below you. Walk around this place, taking notice of all the sounds of relaxation ... those that are close and those that are far away. Notice the soothing fragrances in this safe place ... those that are distinct and those that seem subtle. Be aware of all the safe fragrances. Now notice the temperature and quality of the air ... reach out and touch some of the objects in this place of safety ... notice all the textures. Be aware that anything that is safe can be imported into this place by you. If anything seems unsafe or threatening, allow yourself to send it out and notice how you are able to do this. Feel and appreciate all the relaxing sounds ... assuring smells ... and the sight of safety ... feel it, appreciate it. Take it all in and memorize it so that if someone asked you to draw it at a later date you could do this in great detail... or can call it up at any time (5 – 10 seconds of silence). Also notice how you can begin to move about ... moving about with the feeling of relaxed joyfulness ... relaxed joyfulness ... this is our natural state. Remember what it feels like to be relaxed ... and joyful. Take a moment now to give yourself permission ... full permission to enjoy this state of comfort ... of relaxation ... of peace (be silent for about 10 seconds).

Slowly begin to bring your awareness back into this room, realizing that shortly but not just yet you will open your eyes. Before you do this, realize that you will feel more relaxed and better able to get on with the rest of your day. Make small movements in your fingers and toes ... make small movements in your arms and legs. Whenever you are ready, slowly begin to bring your awareness fully into this room, opening your eyes when you are ready.

Positive Self-Talk and Thought Replacement/Transformation (CR)

Time required: One or more sessions, continuously referring back.
Materials required: List of thinking errors.
Indications for use: Use when the primary need is to enhance cognitive coping skills in the Safety and Stabilization stage of trauma recovery.
Counterindications: Client clearly confused, labile.

This section is strongly influenced by the work developed by Dr. Albert Ellis and Dr. Aaron Beck. These two individuals revolutionized our understanding of errors in thinking and how our thoughts can lead us astray. The power of our internal thoughts can shift us from relative calm to extreme distress. Harnessing our thoughts and challenging where they lead us can be the difference between unsettled internal distress to peace of mind and back. Intentionally learning about our automatic thoughts and challenging the roots and the power of these beliefs can offer us a road to a more settled and calm internal world.

Delivery of Approach

Ten Errors of Thinking and Positive Challenges to Errors in Thinking
Assist your client by reviewing the following Ten Errors of Thinking and how to transform them through positive self-talk and replacement using the Challenges to negative thinking presented later in this section. You can read through the items out loud with your client or have them read them out loud. Give the client time to reflect and comment on each of the Ten Errors of Thinking by asking "Is Error in Thinking something you recognize in yourself and, if yes, how?".

USING THE TOOLS
Ten Errors of Thinking

1. *Exaggeration or minimization.* In the case of exaggerated thinking, small errors may be viewed as major (e.g., I lost my bus ticket – I am the biggest idiot in the world!). Alternatively, in minimization we may undermine our true accomplishments or skills (e.g., "Oh yes, I did get an A on that exam but it was just a fluke").
   Do you do this? If yes, how?
   _____
   _____

2. *All-or-nothing thinking.* This occurs when we fail to see things on the full spectrum of life experiences. For example, a slight inconvenience such as a meal that arrives warm instead of hot results in a declaration that dinner is ruined!
   Do you do this? If yes, how?
   _____
   _____

3. *Overgeneralization.* A single occurrence is viewed as a never-ending negative pattern or prophecy of doom. (e.g., a man's relationship ends and he arrives at the conclusion that all relationships he will develop in the future are doomed to failure).
   Do you do this? If yes, how?
   _____
   _____

4. *Mind reading.* Here, the person believes that their interpretation of what another is thinking must be accurate without fully checking out their own version of the situation (e.g., a woman sees her friend yawning during their conversation and concludes that her friend must think she is a bore; the reality may be that the friend stayed up all night with a sick child).
   Do you do this? If yes, how?
   _____
   _____

5. *Fortune-teller error.* This is an unfortunate tendency to anticipate bad outcomes and then behave as if one's prediction has already occurred (e.g., in anticipation of a job interview the person predicts that they will never get the job – then proceeds to perform poorly during the interview even though they are highly qualified).
   Do you do this? If yes, how?
   _____
   _____

Note: These two pages may be reproduced by the purchaser for clinical use.

From: Anna B. Baranowsky, J. Eric Gentry, & D. Franklin Schultz, *Trauma Practice: Tools for Stabilization and Recovery.* © 2011 Hogrefe Publishing

6. *Should statements.* The individual puts pressure on themselves or others to accomplish something through the utilization of guilt (e.g., "I will disappoint everyone if I don't get this new job"). Conversely, an individual may use guilt to manipulate another (e.g., "If you don't wash my car you do not love me").
Do you do this? If yes, how?

_____

_____

7. *Labeling.* The person uses name-calling or negative labels to describe errors made by themselves or others instead of simply describing the mistake (e.g., "I'm *totally useless* for forgetting to take the muffins out of the oven in time").
Do you do this? If yes, how?

_____

_____

8. *Personalization.* Taking personal responsibility for a negative outcome that the person is not entirely responsible for (e.g., a person may say, "I lost the game" when they were playing a team sport and therefore only one player in a group). Do you do this? If yes, how?

_____

_____

9. *Emotional reasoning.* This is the act of believing that because you feel very badly about something, every one else must be equally devastated or disgusted by the event (e.g., "I lost my new team jacket and feel awful – I have let everyone down by my actions and they must feel devastated about this loss").
Do you do this? If yes, how?

_____

_____

10. *Disqualifying the positive.* Here, positive outcomes, accomplishments, and experiences are discounted while the meaning of negative events are elevated in one's view (e.g., one negative comment is taken much more seriously than many examples of positive feedback). The constructive criticism one receives is extremely important, whereas positive feedback is quickly forgotten.
Do you do this? If yes, how?

_____

_____

Note: These two pages may be reproduced by the purchaser for clinical use.

In the acronym CHANGES, each letter stands for one challenge to the Ten Errors in Thinking outlined above. There are seven items in this section to help you challenge negative thoughts and improve internal dialogue. Work with your client to review all the items below and then give homework sheets "Reflection Sheet #1 and #2".

USING THE TOOLS
CHANGES – Positive Challenges to Errors in Thinking

1. *C – Concretize:* Arriving at exaggerated statements of events such as "it will never get better" or "this is devastating" are the result of thinking errors like exaggerated thinking or overgeneralization. Questioning the statement of belief can bring a bit of reality back into the picture. An exaggerated statement such as those above could be challenged as follows: "Will it really never get better?" or "Is it so devastating that we should call an ambulance, police, or the Red Cross?"
2. *H – Humor:* Using humor to defuse our thinking errors can be very effective. Although we are able to laugh at comedy shows depicting events very familiar to us, when we are personally involved we become unable to see the humor. The goal in using humor is to step back, view the situation with detachment, and search for the humor in the event.
3. *A – Alternatives:* The use of alternatives broadens our currently narrow view on an event. One can challenge virtually all the errors in thinking utilizing this approach. Initially, the goal is simply to identify alternatives to the current belief. You may be unable to believe the alternative, but it starts to broaden your thoughts and that is the goal. You may think "my roommate hates me," or alternatively you may challenge this with "my roommate and I are different people and enjoy different things."
4. *N – Normal Others:* The task here is to identify others whom you admire and feel are managing their lives well. Then, when confronted with an error in your own thinking, you ask yourself "What would X say about this?" or "How would X handle this?"
5. *G – Good for Me:* Use this strategy whenever your thoughts are negative or unhelpful. For example, if I have some document to review and conclude that "I will never get this done," the challenging question would be "Is this thought helpful in achieving my goal of reviewing the document?" Of course, the answer would be no. The next question would be "What thought would help me achieve my goal?" This might be "If I put aside a little time each day this week I will get this work completed." In this way, we find thoughts that are good for us and useful in helping us arrive at our desired outcome.
6. *E – Evidence:* Use this when you get stuck on thoughts that arrive at conclusions without sufficient evidence (e.g., "I'm going to die," in response to anxious feelings associated with a racing heartbeat). Challenge yourself with evidence-seeking questions, such as "Have you died in the past when you had these feelings?"
7. *S – So What?* Use this when thoughts are upsetting but you are not certain what error in thinking you have made. Challenge your negative thoughts or conclusions with "So what?" For example, you may be worried about an upcoming meeting and conclude, "I will make a fool of myself!" Challenge your belief by saying "So what?" If you respond with another negative thought like "It would be so embarrassing," again say "So what?" Keep challenging yourself with "So what?" until negative thoughts are exhausted.

These seven thought challenges are designed to broaden and improve your own thought patterns so as to include a more useful, nourishing, and sustainable internal dialogue. Run through one or more of the challenges above whenever you have errors in thinking. Continue the process until the errors reduce or are, at the very least, exposed.

Note: This page may be reproduced by the purchaser for clinical use.

From: Anna B. Baranowsky, J. Eric Gentry, & D. Franklin Schultz, *Trauma Practice: Tools for Stabilization and Recovery.* © 2011 Hogrefe Publishing

Use Reflection Sheets #1 and #2 to assist in externalizing negative thoughts and challenging them.

USING THE TOOLS
Reflection Sheet #1

Date	Situation	Automatic thought	Feeling	Error type
Example 05/08/02	Job interview	I'll blow it. They will think I'm ridiculous.	Panic, hopelessness	Fortune teller, Mind reading

Note: This page may be reproduced by the purchaser for clinical use.

From: Anna B. Baranowsky, J. Eric Gentry, & D. Franklin Schultz, *Trauma Practice: Tools for Stabilization and Recovery.* © 2011 Hogrefe Publishing

Reflection Sheet #2

Date: _____

Situation	(What were you doing)? Example: Preparing for a job interview.
Feelings	(Describe and rate 1 – 10 where 1 = no distress to 10 = extreme distress) Example: Panic, Hopeless, Fearful – *Rating* = 8
Trigger thoughts (images)	(What was going through your mind just prior to the bad feelings? What other thoughts or images came up?) Example: I'll blow it. They will think I'm ridiculous.
How to make changes to trigger thoughts	Concretize: "Shall we alert the Red Cross?" Humor: "How can I see the humor in this?" Alternatives: "Can I see this in a more positive light or just differently?" Normal Others: "What would X think about this?" or "How would X handle this?" Good for Me: "Is this thought good for me or useful?" Evidence: "Is there enough evidence for me to believe it is 100% true? How so? How not?" So What: And if all else fails, "SO WHAT!"
Balancing thoughts	(Phrase a "neutral or balanced" statement to replace the error in thinking.) (Next, rate how much you believe the new statement from 0 to 100%.) Example: I will do my best at this interview and learn from my experience. *Rating* = 75%
Rate feeling now	(Describe and rate 1 – 10 where 1 = no distress to 10 = extreme distress) Example: Panic, Hopeless, Fearful *Rating* = 3

Note: This page may be reproduced by the purchaser for clinical use.

From: Anna B. Baranowsky, J. Eric Gentry, & D. Franklin Schultz, *Trauma Practice: Tools for Stabilization and Recovery.* © 2011 Hogrefe Publishing

Flashback Journal (R – RE)

Time required: Approximately 10 – 20 minutes, continuously referring back.
Materials required: Journal.
Indications for use: Use when the primary need is to enhance cognitive and behavioral coping skills in the Safety and Stabilization stage of trauma recovery.
Counterindications: If client is overwhelmed by events and unable to self-soothe.

Delivery of Approach

The following journal format is useful as a functional analysis of triggers and symptoms. Column labels are self-explanatory. Have the client note specific symptoms when they occur. Then have them identify what was occurring at the moment that may have triggered the symptom. Next, have them identify the event with which it may be associated and make an estimated SUDs level. Have them use self-soothing skills and reestimate their SUDs level.

USING THE TOOLS
Flashback Journal

Symptom	Trigger	Memory	SUDs	Self-soothing skill(s) used	SUDs

Note: This page may be reproduced by the purchaser for clinical use.

From: Anna B. Baranowsky, J. Eric Gentry, & D. Franklin Schultz, *Trauma Practice: Tools for Stabilization and Recovery.* © 2011 Hogrefe Publishing

Thought-Stopping (R – RE – CR)

Time required: 5 minutes.
Materials required: None.
Indications for use: Use when the primary need is to enhance cognitive coping skills in the Safety and Stabilization stage of trauma recovery.
Counterindications: If client is unable to self-soothe, has low expectation for success, is labile, and/or has low self-esteem.

Thought-stopping is an exercise that has been used with varying degrees of success by many individuals. We will cover it briefly in this section, mostly because it is a commonly used exercise and is therefore worth touching on, if only just to familiarize yourself. Thought-stopping is not a technique that we have found to achieve consistent success, but when it works it can be very useful. Unfortunately, it creates an uncomfortably stressful feeling for many individuals and frequently results in a feeling of failure. Nonetheless, we will consider it primarily for historical value and the recognition that, with an open mind, we can revisit interventions with the goal of efficacy identification.

Delivery of Approach

The exercise can be taught in several ways. The two most popular methods are described in this section. Both require a sharp response to any negative thoughts or images. The goal is to diminish or stop the negative images or thoughts, at least temporarily. The client begins by recognizing a negative thought or image that has intruded into their minds. The client is instructed first to yell out loud "Stop!" thus sending the message to one's own mind to end one's focus on the negative thought or image. Eventually, the loud stop message is "screamed" within one's own mind. Alternatively, the individual has an elastic band on their wrist. Whenever a negative thought or image intrudes they are instructed to snap the band. In both cases, it is believed that the thought or image will diminish over time. In some cases this does occur. However, in many cases the feedback is inconsistent. Many individuals feel that the solution is very temporary and leaves them feeling distracted rather than relieved. In the following exercise we will explore why this occurs and how it is often better to offer gentle solutions, challenges to negative beliefs, and a commitment to resolution time.

Buddha's Trick (R – CR)

Time required: 5 minutes.
Materials required: None.
Indications for use: Use when the primary need is to enhance cognitive coping skills in the Safety and Stabilization stage of trauma recovery.
Counterindications: Client clearly confused, unable to concentrate, actively dissociating.

This is an awareness technique to assist clients by improving their understanding of the necessity for processing time and the level of energy required for suppression. Many people who have been exposed to traumatic events attempt to "push bad thoughts out of their minds." In significant numbers, this approach tends to result in the unfortunate outcome of posttrauma symptoms (i.e., intrusive thoughts, poor sleep, anxious feelings, and avoidance). By refusing to think about difficult events, we fail to establish a complete narrative, make sense of our experiences, desensitize through exposure, and recognize that we are now safe. Baer (2001) provides an excellent illustration of this technique in *The Imp of the Mind* (pp. 95–99).

When we are feeling very badly about something that has occurred or that we worry might occur, we sometimes make a strong effort to "suppress" our thoughts, feelings, and memories associated with the disturbing recollection. Many research studies show that this type of thought suppression does not work. In addition, it uses a large amount of energy to keep thoughts out of our mind and is therefore exhausting. It also increases the fear factor as we are hiding this thing from our thoughts, reducing our ability to review and resolve our feelings and thus making it seem even more unbearable than it is. Recall someone saying to you that something terrible has happened and then not telling you right away what it is. Your mind arrives at a conclusion that is even worse than the actual reality, in most cases.

Delivery of Approach

Thought Exercise

1. Instruct the individual to think of a "stone Buddha" or any other non-anxiety producing object (e.g., pink elefant, puppy dog) for 1 minute, keeping their mind as focused as possible during this time. If at any time they lose their focus, they are to lift a finger to alert both themselves and you that they have lost their focus. Now discuss what this exercise was like, what they observed, and how much energy it took to keep their mind focused.
2. Next, the individual is instructed to keep "stone Buddhas" out of their mind for a full minute. Again, they are to lift a finger every time "stone Buddha" comes into the mind. When the minute is over they are given time to reflect on the difficulty of this exercise and the amount of energy it takes to keep the mind focused.
3. Now they are asked to notice if "stone Buddhas" come to mind at an even greater rate than prior to thought suppression. This is called the *rebound effect* and is also noted in a number of research studies. These studies show that the use of suppression results in traumatic memories surfacing more often and more vigorously than prior to suppression. This is a good way to teach clients that, although they are trying to suppress traumatic memories, the use of suppression often makes it more difficult to manage trauma memory intrusions when they surface and that suppression is simply not an effective method of managing historical trauma.
4. Explain this phenomenon to the individual so they understand the importance of reflection and resolution, as opposed to the tendency to want to suppress our negative thoughts, feelings, memories, or fears.

This is an extremely useful approach to preparing the individual for trauma review and reducing treatment resistance as the individual begins to recognize that he or she is continually thinking about the feared event because suppression does not work efficiently and is likely the reason for ongoing feeling of distress. This exercise is also a practical clarification as to why Thought-Stopping is frequently unsatisfying for individuals seeking relief of trauma-loaded thoughts.

4. Behavior

There is a tendency to believe that behaviors are nothing more than the end result of our body and mind working together to accomplish an end. This is seen as a one-way flow of information from inside to outside. However, the truth is that information flows both ways. How clients behave is how they will begin to see and understand themselves. If they act in unsafe ways or perform less-than-useful behaviors to manage their anxiety, they often believe that they are helpless to do anything else. In turn, if they act in ways that are more useful in keeping themselves safe and less anxious, they will come to believe they have the power to change. Many times, clients do not have the skills or experience necessary to create more useful behaviors. This section provides techniques to aid in the creation of new options.

Rituals (R – CR)

Time required: One session or more.
Materials required: Paper and pencil/contract.
Indications for use: Use when the primary need is to enhance

Ritualistic methods for safety and stabilization can vary widely. The key is to create a form of practice or ceremony that reinforces the individual's sense of reassurance, safety, or security. One meaningful ritual is to have a "marriage" ceremony with oneself. This ritual effectively strengthens the internal tie by affirming the individual's commitment for personal responsibility and fully empowers the person to act on their own best behalf. If things are not going well or goals have been set, they must look to themselves to move their lives forward in the desired

behavioral coping skills in the Safety and Stabilization stage of trauma recovery.
Counterindications: Depends on the ritual selected.

direction. This takes an act of will, but it is much more likely that we will achieve our greatest hopes and dreams if we take full responsibility for these dreams. After all, who else is as fully informed of what we truly wish from life if not ourselves?

Delivery of Approach

The ceremony is to be orchestrated in the vision of the individual. This can be completed alone or in the company of trusted counselors or friends/family. In one example, the individual chose to complete the ritual alone. Candles were lit, paint and paper was available for creative expression, a colorful silk robe was worn and meaningful music was played. The individual wrote their wishes for the future and their commitment to themselves. They wrote a "self-marriage" ceremony in which they made a strong and earnest vow to "care for themselves in a manner that met their inner desires, hopes and dreams." In effect, this ceremony was a joyous occasion of personal commitment to the future and self-support. The individual came to the conclusion that if they treated themselves in this manner they would have nothing to feel disappointed about, and if they did not they would have no one to blame other than themselves.

Examples:
Below you will find a list of sample rituals, many of which have been described in trauma practice workshops that we offer nationally and internationally. This list offers very brief descriptions of different rituals that can be undertaken by individuals or groups. The idea is to let one's imagination open up to the possibility of a meaningful expression of self.

- Perform a ceremony alone or with others to celebrate one's earlier life and then a ceremony to celebrate a "rebirth to a new way of living" – one that allows for healthier choices and new opportunities.
- Burn a list of harmful traumatic memories.
- Collect photos of earlier life to use as a point of reference for moving forward in life.
- Construct a collage to make a representation of internal experiences.
- Attach objects for healing or names of survivors to helium balloons and symbolically release objects/persons to freedom along with the balloon.
- Prepare a shrine or memory collection of grief to help maintain a connection with a person who has died.
- Write a letter to a person who has died or one whom you have unfinished business with (letters do not need to be sent).
- Conduct services of thanksgiving or reconciliation.
- Maintain a journal.
- Perform positive daily affirmations.
- Videotape "survival and resiliency" experiences of survivors to share with future survivors.
- Construct hope quilts from squares made by survivors.
- Construct a safety collage filled with reassuring and comforting images.
- Prepare certificates of success with positive comments from others.
- Paint rocks with meaningful symbols and display them in prominent places as reminders of recovery.
- Make a self-care box filled with examples of things to do to feel good; when not feeling well, pick something out of the box.

USING THE TOOLS
Rituals

Because there are many possible safety and stabilization rituals, we offer you a place to recall and collect or imagine rituals that may be meaningful for you or your clients. Using the space available, describe rituals for which you wish to keep a record for future use.

_____

_____

_____

_____

_____

_____

_____

_____

_____

_____

_____

_____

_____

_____

_____

_____

_____

_____

_____

_____

Note: This page may be reproduced by the purchaser for clinical use.

From: Anna B. Baranowsky, J. Eric Gentry, & D. Franklin Schultz, *Trauma Practice: Tools for Stabilization and Recovery.* © 2011 Hogrefe Publishing

Contract for Safety and Self-Care (R – CR)

Time required: One session or more.
Materials required: Paper and pencil/contract.
Indications for use: Use when the primary need is to enhance behavioral coping skills in the Safety and Stabilization stage of trauma recovery.
Counterindications: None.

Delivery of Approach

Another approach is to make a concrete commitment or contract in writing to move toward healing. An example of this follows.

USING THE TOOLS
Contract for Safety and Self-Care

Name: _____ Date: _____

Safety Goal Area: _____ (My goal)

I care about myself and am committed to my healing. I realize that, to be well, I have to make changes in my life and the way I live it. By making these changes, no matter how small, I am affirming my choice to become the person I want to be.

I want (to):
_____
_____

(My goal)

I will prove to myself that I am committed to becoming my best self by completing the following behavioral objectives (tiny achievable steps):

Self-Care:
_____
_____

Connection with Others:
_____
_____

Self-Soothing Skills Acquisition:
_____
_____

I will complete these affirmations of myself on or before: _____

Signature: _____ Date: _____

Witness : _____ Date: _____

Note: This page may be reproduced by the purchaser for clinical use.

From: Anna B. Baranowsky, J. Eric Gentry, & D. Franklin Schultz, *Trauma Practice: Tools for Stabilization and Recovery.* © 2011 Hogrefe Publishing

Safety Net Plan (R – CR)

Time required: One session.
Materials required: Paper and pencil.
Indications for use: Use when the primary need is to enhance behavioral coping skills in the Safety and Stabilization stage of trauma recovery.
Counterindications: None.

Delivery of Approach

A Safety Net Plan is a personalized master plan of what you can do when you feel overwhelmed, out of control, helpless, and/or at a loss of what you need to do to find your own safety again. Remember, it is always better to plan ahead than to have to act without a plan in a crisis.

USING THE TOOLS
Safety Net Plan

This document is to help you be better prepared for difficult times when they arise throughout the course of your treatment. It will help you become more self-sufficient and resilient to the daily stressors of being a survivor.

Self-Help Capacities

You have managed many difficult situations in the past successfully and used different abilities and techniques to do so. Let us inventory some of these abilities and self-soothing techniques (activities that help you calm down) so that you can refer back to them when necessary. Remember, you might want to use one technique after the other until you find one that works.

Self-soothing techniques (e.g., talking positively with your self, taking a bath, writing, reading):

1. _____
2. _____
3. _____

Abilities used in the past to manage difficult situations: (e.g., creativity, accepting help, courage, tenacity):

1. _____
2. _____
3. _____

Informal Support

Below, list names of friends and family members you feel free to contact when you need help. Establish that your supporters are willing to help (for your own assurance) and tell them how they can best assist you when you are in a crisis. They will not know what you do and do not need unless you tell them. Please make a check mark next to their name after you have talked with them about their willingness to help. Different people have different strengths and might be better at helping in one situation than in another.

Remember, it is the quality – not the quantity – of your supporters that counts.

Supporter's name	Phone numbers	Supporter's helping strengths
1.		
2.		
3.		

Note: This page may be reproduced by the purchaser for clinical use.

From: Anna B. Baranowsky, J. Eric Gentry, & D. Franklin Schultz, *Trauma Practice: Tools for Stabilization and Recovery.* © 2011 Hogrefe Publishing

Timed and Metered Expression Strategies (R – RE)

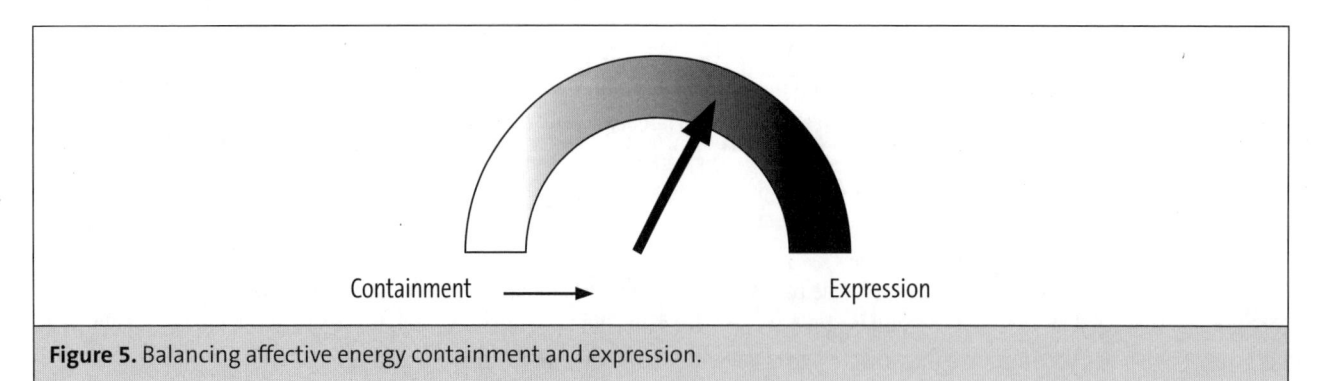

Figure 5. Balancing affective energy containment and expression.

Time required: 5–30 minutes.
Materials required: None/pillows/paper.
Indications for use: Use when the primary need is to enhance cognitive, emotional, and behavioral coping skills in the Safety and Stabilization stage of trauma recovery.
Counterindications: Emotionally labile, actively dissociating or dissociates during exercise.

Sometimes, when working with trauma survivors, the survivors become overwhelmed by the affective energy associated with a flashback or abreaction and they are unable to self-soothe or contain this energy. In these situations, it is helpful to guide the client through some highly structured exercises that allow them to express, or bleed-off, some of the energy associated with this abreaction. The metaphor of allowing some of the steam to escape a pressure cooker is helpful in understanding this process.

We believe that these expressive strategies should *only* be used when (a) the client is unable to successfully self-soothe, ground, and contain this energy, or (b) the client has articulated the desire to work with the expression of this negative affect.

Delivery of Approach

The goal of this work is to develop a safe, controlled expression and resolution of these negative feelings and not to trigger a full-blown abreaction. This exercise should begin and end with the client being in control. There are several ways in which this can be achieved:

Sounds
1. Take a SUDs level (0–10). This will probably be in the 8–10 range because it should only be employed when the client is overwhelmed with affect.
2. Instruct the client, "Notice all the sounds and words that you currently 'hear' in your abdomen and chest."
3. "Now, for the next one minute of clock time, I'd like for you to express these sounds and words."
4. Simply witness and support your client with minimal encouragement (e.g., "that's right") during the expression of these sounds and words.
5. At the end of one minute, stop the client. Take a SUDs level. Ask the client to discuss with you what has happened and describe that experience.
6. Ask the client if they experienced enough relief to continue with their work, or whether they need to further express these feelings. If they need additional expression, ask them for an amount of time that they would like to be engaged in the expression exercise (e.g., 1, 2, 5 minutes) and indicate when to begin.
7. After the negotiated time is completed, no matter if they are right in the middle of expression, stop this process! Take a SUDs level. Discuss with them their experiences. Renego-

tiate for more time, if necessary, until they have achieved relief from the *overwhelming* energy of the abreaction. (*Note:* They may not have reached a level of comfort, but will probably reach a level of manageability. This will probably be a SUDs level of 4–6.)
8. The clinician should take great pains to point out to the client that they were able to move into and out of this intense affect and remain in control and did not become overwhelmed. This is important *experiential* learning for the client that helps them dissolve their fear of strong emotion.
9. Assist your client with the use of a self-soothing technique to calm and soften any residual affect.

Pillows
1. Arrange large pile of cushions in the lap of the client.
2. Take a SUDs level. Next, ask the client for the number (between 5 and 10) that reflects how many times they believe they need to hit the pillows for the negative energy of their affect to be discharged and for the SUDs to reach a level of 5.
3. Instruct the client, "Now put your two hands together, raise them over your head, and strike the pillows/cushions as hard as you can, making a sound, from your belly, on each downward stroke."
4. Stop them after they have struck the pillows/cushions their negotiated number of times. Take a SUDs level.
5. Discuss with them this experience and ask them to indicate whether they are able to orient sufficiently to utilize self-soothing skills to manage affect, or if they need to utilize more expression.
6. If they indicate the need for more expression, take a SUDs level, negotiate a number of "hits," and then repeat steps 3–5 above.
7. The clinician should take great pains to point out to the client that they were able to move into and out of this intense affect and remain in control and did not become overwhelmed. This is important *experiential* learning for the client that helps them to dissolve their fear of strong emotion.
8. Assist the client with the use of a self-soothing technique to calm and soften any residual affect.

Tearing Paper
Using the same steps above, the tearing of paper can be substituted for hitting pillows. Be sure to encourage the client to express visceral "sounds" while tearing.

Crying
For clients who articulate a fear of crying, but who also have demonstrated the need for the expression of this affect, a timed experience of crying can be helpful. Using the same steps delineated above, ask the client to select a period of time that they will allow themselves to fully express grief, loss, and sadness by crying (2–5 minutes is recommended for the first time). The clinician should "bear witness" with minimal encouragement of this process and should stop and process at the appointed elapsed time. Renegotiate for additional time, as needed. Be sure to include plenty of time for processing, discussion, and self-soothing.

Note: Richard Kluft (personal communication, 1994) has articulated the "rule of thirds" when working with expression and abreaction. This rule suggests that if the client and clinician are unable to address this difficult material within the first two-thirds of the session time, it should not be approached or attempted in the last third of the session. The risk of an incomplete session that could potentially retraumatize the client is too great. Utilize a grounding, anxiety reduction (self-soothing), or containment strategy if you have entered this last third of the session with your client and these painful affects surface.

5. Emotion/Relation

One of the most damaging long-term effects of trauma is the manner in which it constricts the survivor's ability to feel a full range of emotion and connect to other people. This is true whether the trauma is inflicted by another person or experienced as an accident or an act of nature. Fear and anxiety create such a high state of arousal that emotions are shut down. This occurs because the areas in the brain responsible for emotions are directly linked to the survival routines. If the trauma is abuse, the violation of trust makes it difficult to connect to others for fear of being harmed. Traumatic experiences can lead to intrusive fear that is overwhelming. This often results in constriction of emotion, feelings of powerlessness, and eventual withdrawal, and makes it difficult to connect to others. Learning to feel and learning to connect with others are powerful healing agents that mitigate the effects of trauma. This is a process that requires all the skills of self-soothing because the overwhelming feelings happen so quickly. This section provides techniques useful to that end.

Transitional Objects (R)

Time required: Minimal.
Materials required: Varies.
Indications for use: Use when the primary need is to enhance emotional coping skills in the Safety and Stabilization stage of trauma recovery.
Counterindications: None.

Transitional objects are representations of supportive persons, places, things, or memories. These may take the form of soothing objects, such as a blanket that reminds the individual of safe moments in a loving care-provider's arms, a stuffed toy given by a cherished friend, or a pebble picked up at a beach while enjoying much-needed rest and relaxation.

Delivery of Approach

A transitional object can be anything. The key is what it represents for the individual and whether they can use the object to anchor safety, security, comfort, and relaxation for themselves. One object may suffice or several may be selected collectively or individually to create a sense of grounded comfort for the individual. Objects can be identified through a visualization exercise similar to the Safe-Place Visualization exercise described earlier or simply through self-awareness by asking "Is there something, some object that represents comfort to you?" If the individual is not able to identify anything, it may be planted through the Safe-Place Visualization by adding a suggestion of finding an object that represents safety, security, and comfort during the imaging process. In this way, the individual is able to identify an object that they can invest with meaning.

Support Systems (R – CR)

Time required: 30 minutes.
Materials required: Paper and pencil.
Indications for use: Use when the primary need is to enhance emotional coping skills in the Safety and Stabilization stage of trauma recovery.
Counterindications: Actively dissociating or dissociates during exercise.

Research indicates that social support is a buffer to the struggles of everyday life. It becomes even more important when we face tough times and trauma. The following exercise is an imagery exercise to assist individuals in identifying social supports that can create the basis of this powerful buffer. In the following exercise, we encourage individuals to find their own "Committee of Comfort and Support."

Delivery of Approach

Committee of Comfort and Support
Invite the client to find a comfortable position, begin to relax, close their eyes, and focus inwardly. Ask the individual to imagine the "safe place and safe object" they visited and identi-

fied in earlier safety exercises (if they have done so – otherwise return to earlier exercises to accomplish this first). Encourage them to recall and describe the safety object and use it to guide them right back to their safe place. Ask them to see all that they would see in their safe place, hear what they would hear, smell what they would smell, and sense or feel what they would sense or feel in their place of safety.

Remind your client to reclaim the feelings of safety, comfort, and reassurance associated with their safety object and place in whatever way is meaningful to them.

Instruct the client at this time to "begin to call in toward you all the people in your life who you feel would be good members of a Committee of Comfort and Support. These people could be present and involved in your life right now, or helpful in the past but no longer in your life at this time for any reason. They might be imagined or ideal persons, or those who you knew and are no longer alive. These would be people who would not judge you, and who you feel completely safe with and supported by. Call them in one by one, becoming very aware of who they are what they look like, their names."

Encourage the individual to make the members of their team as concrete as possible. Remind them that "these are the figures who you can call on when you are needing support in your everyday life ... you can draw on these members for wisdom, emotional support, play time, etc. Review the members of your team and ask any members you no longer feel completely supported by and safe with to leave. Watch as they leave the circle, urged only with a polite but firm statement that it is time for them to leave now. Once again invite any new members in to take the places of those you have asked to leave."

Ask your client to lift one finger to let you know when their committee is formed.

Now have the individual focus inwardly again. Suggest that they imagine a member of their committee moving toward them and sharing words of support and genuine care with them. Have them allow the internal dialogue to remain positive and nurturing.

Inform the client that you will be silent for 1 minute of clock time while they have this positive internal dialogue.

When the minute is over, ask them to slowly bring their attention back into the room and open their eyes when they are ready.

Provide a sheet for the client to write on and instruct them to "Write out all the names of the committee members on this sheet."

Process the experience. Ask the client "What effect did this exercise have on you?"

USING THE TOOLS
Safe Place Imagery: My Committee of Comfort and Support

This exercise is designed to help you "fire" the "negativity committee" that creates the nonstop chatter, criticism, and self-depreciation in your mind. This exercise will help you to replace this negativity with support, comfort, and affirmation.

Write out the names of all the people from your life who have contributed to your health or esteem, and/or who you have admired. These can be real people with whom you have had relationships in the past. They can be important people from your life with whom you are no longer in contact. They can be people from public life, historical or present, that have contributed to your worth. They can be religious leaders or icons. They can be imaginary or real. There is no limit to who or how many people can comprise your Committee of Comfort and Support. Please list your committee members on the sheet below.

Remember it is the quality – not the quantity – of persons you list that counts.

My Committee

1.	11.
2.	12.
3.	13.
4.	14.
5.	15.
6.	16.
7.	17.
8.	18.
9.	19.
10.	20.

Note: This page may be reproduced by the purchaser for clinical use.

From: Anna B. Baranowsky, J. Eric Gentry, & D. Franklin Schultz, *Trauma Practice: Tools for Stabilization and Recovery.* © 2011 Hogrefe Publishing

Drawing Icon and Envelope (Emotional Containment) (R – RE – CR)

Time required: 10–30 minutes.
Materials required: Papers, colored markers, envelope, and stapler.
Indications for use: Use when the primary need is to enhance emotional coping skills in the Safety and Stabilization stage of trauma recovery.
Counterindications: Actively dissociating or dissociates during exercise.

The capacity to contain posttraumatic images, feelings, and thoughts is a crucial skill that must be developed with a client before they can truly confront and resolve a traumatic memory from a perspective of choice. If a client is unable to set aside incomplete therapeutic work on their traumatic memories and successfully reenter normal life and its demands, then the client runs a high risk of becoming retraumatized by the work of therapy. With this in mind, it is important that the trauma therapist develop, with their clients, some effective strategies for containing these incomplete or fragmented memories, thoughts, and feelings relative to traumatic experiences.

We have found an art therapy technique to be very helpful in developing this capacity for containment. We utilize this technique often when the time of a session has nearly elapsed and the client is still deeply engrossed in the traumatic material. This method allows the client to "package" these difficult images, feelings, and thoughts for work in a later session.

Home Use

Instructing the client in the use a variation of this method can be very helpful for the individual who is experiencing frequent disruptive flashbacks in their day-to-day life. Ask them to briefly draw an icon (less than 5 minutes) of the memory, flashback, or painful images and then put it inside an envelope and address it to their therapist's office. They should also be instructed to mail this "letter" as soon as possible after completing the drawing. The client should be informed that the drawing will be kept safely in their file and the therapist will address these drawings with the client at their next meeting. They will become part of the trauma treatment plan.

Delivery of Approach

1. Using colored pencils/markers, ask the client to draw a *symbol* that represents the memory, along with its feelings, images, and thoughts. This should be only an abstract symbol, and not a drawing of the event(s). No more than 5 minutes should be allowed for this drawing.
2. When the client has completed the drawing, ask them to place it inside a manila envelope and seal the envelope.
3. Hand the client a stapler and instruct them to put as many staples in the envelope as necessary to contain this material for a time that it can be addressed in the future. Allow them as many staples as they wish.
4. Ask them to write the title of this memory/material on the outside of the envelope.
5. Tell the client that you will keep this envelope, along with all its negative thoughts and feelings, secure inside their case file. It will remain safely contained there until the client is ready to work again toward the resolution of this memory.
6. Inform the client that if they think of the memory in the future, they need not return to the helpless and overwhelming feelings present during the traumatic event. Instead they can recall that this memory is safe in their therapist's office.
7. Encourage the client to utilize grounding/self-soothing strategies to regain full control before leaving the office (asking the client to count backwards from 100 by 7s is an excellent exercise to help engage neocortical functioning and reorient to the present).

Internal Vault (Emotional Containment) (R – RE – CR)

Time required: 5–10 minutes.
Materials required: None.
Indications for use: Use when the primary need is to enhance emotional coping skills in the

Delivery of Approach

This technique, while drawing from hypnotherapy, can be utilized in a variety of contexts. Simply, it is assisting the client in developing an "internal vault" into which they can place uncomfortable memories, feelings, thoughts, and other negative artifacts of traumatic memories.

Safety and Stabilization stage of trauma recovery.
Counterindications: Actively dissociating or dissociates during exercise.

This technique works well with clients who have the capacity for dissociation. One elegant strategy that includes this technique is to assist the client with visualizing a "steel vault that has a locked door" when doing the Safe Place Visualization exercise. This allows the client to "store" these negative experiences, temporarily, between sessions and allows them to attend to the demands of their daily life without becoming overwhelmed by the traumatic memories.

Positive Hope Box (R – RE – CR)

Time required: 5 minutes.
Materials required: Paper and pencil, small box.
Indications for use: Use when the primary need is to enhance emotional coping skills in the Safety and Stabilization stage of trauma recovery.
Counterindications: None.

Delivery of Approach

Most of us have heard people tell of using cigar boxes in which they write out their hopes, dreams, fears, etc., and then pray for a higher power or God to "take care of it" for them. Being careful to remain sensitive to each individual's spirituality, we have utilized a variation of this folk technique. We ask trauma survivors to decorate a box (cigar boxes work well) with drawings and clippings from magazines that depict images of healing. With this done, we ask them to draw pictures or write words that represent all the overwhelming aspects of their trauma memories and their current life. If they are spiritual, we suggest that they allow their higher power to intervene on their behalf in these areas. If this is not appropriate for the client, we ask that they pick one or two of these areas to bring each week to work on in therapy and to build a ritual that indicates completion (for the individual) when one of these areas has been successfully resolved.

Section 3
Trauma Memory Processing

In the words of Ingrid Collins, a British consulting psychologist,
"When you give patients time and attention, they can relax into healing."
Carl Honore, *In Praise of Slow* (2004)

Reconnection

TRAUMA MEMORY PROCESSING

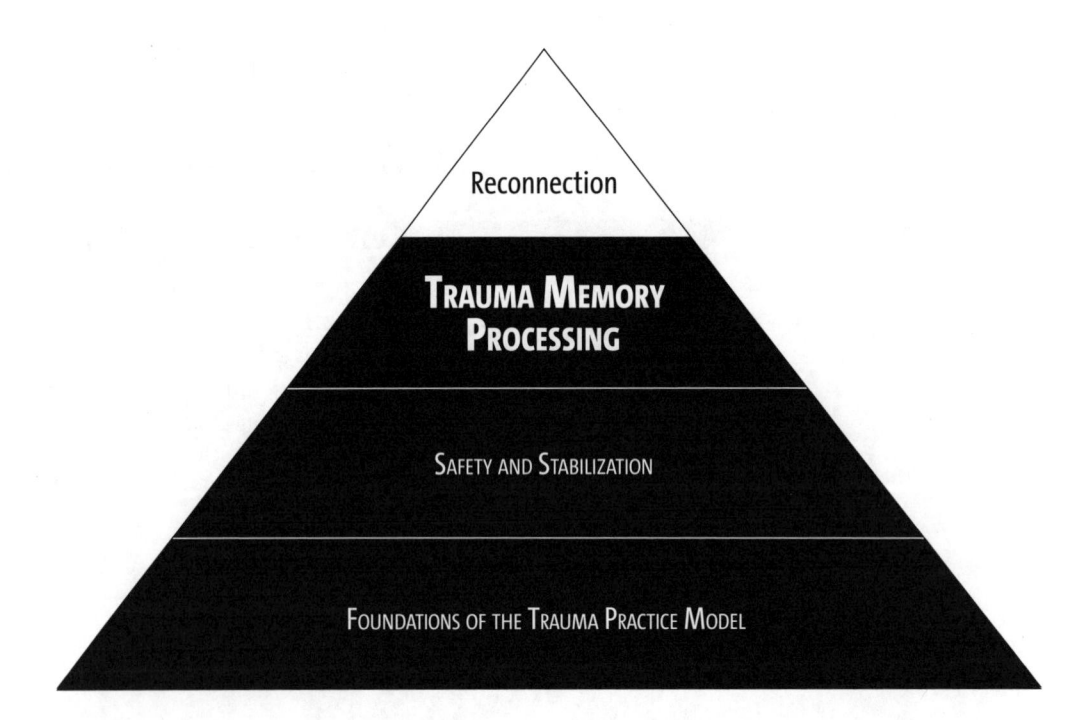

SAFETY AND STABILIZATION

FOUNDATIONS OF THE TRAUMA PRACTICE MODEL

1. Body
  Titration Part II: Braking and Acceleration (RE)
  Layering (RE – CR)
  Comfort in One Part (RE)
  A Time-Line Approach (RE – CR)
  Biofeedback (R – RE – CR)

2. Cognition
  Downward Arrow Technique (RE – CR)
  Cognitive Continuum (CR)
  Calculating True Danger (CR)
  Looped Tape Scripting (RE – CR)
  Cognitive Processing Therapy (RE – CR)
  A Story-Book Approach (RE – CR)
  A Written Narrative Approach (RE – CR)

3. Behavior
  Behavior Change Rehearsal Exercise (RE – CR)
  Skills Building Methods (CR)
  Imaginal and In-Vivo Exposure (RE)
  Stress Inoculation Training (RE – CR)
  Systematic Desensitization (RE)

4. Emotion/Relation
  Learning to Be Sad (CR)
  Assertiveness Training (CR)

In this section, we cover Trauma Memory Processing, moving into the body of the Trauma Practice work that allows the client to process and work through unresolved traumatic memories. As mentioned previously, we believe there are three active and necessary ingredients for the effective treatment of trauma. These include relaxation and exposure (reciprocal inhibition) and cognitive restructuring. From the physiological perspective, this can be understood as facilitating the natural process of the neocortex without triggering the survival routines that shut down processing and might potentially result in retraumatization. In each of the techniques that follow, notice how this could be happening. While the techniques may have different means of maintaining relaxation, remembering, and processing the memory, each involves one or more of relaxation, exposure, and cognitive restructuring.

Much of the work in this section can be linked back to the Trigger List developed in Phase I, Safety and Stabilization. Progress can also be checked by reflecting on changes in the Trigger List SUDs ratings. It is not unusual to see a SUDs reduction when one significant trauma memory is resolved. Returning to the Trigger List gives us a map to review progress over time. Remember, now that you are moving into the Trauma Memory Processing stage of this work you will need to ensure that your client is emotionally, physiologically, and cognitively prepared to move forward into Phase II.

Start by reviewing the essential criterion required to signal client readiness to move to Phase II, Trauma Memory Processing work.

Five Criteria:
1. Resolve danger.
2. Distinguish Am Safe vs. Feel Safe.
3. Develop self-soothe and self-rescue skills.
4. Practice-demo self-rescue.
5. Negotiate contract and informed consent.

1. Body

The physiological key to successful recovery is relaxation. The goal is to have the event fully processed by the neocortex. As anxiety levels go up, processing goes down due to the mechanisms previously discussed. Teaching clients to be aware of their own anxiety levels and providing them with tools to titrate and lower their anxiety will facilitate this process. The techniques discussed in this section will provide a variety of methods to accomplish that task.

Titration Part II: Braking and Acceleration (RE)

Braking and Acceleration is a necessary skill when conducting trauma work. This enables the client to begin their work with the knowledge that they can stop whenever needed. In Part I of Braking and Acceleration we began to look at initial skills through the lens of Safety and Stabilization. Now we begin to look at useful methods that can be implemented during the core of Traumatic Memory Processing. In this way, clients can begin their processing with the assurance that they can always put the brakes on. They can maintain some control over their experience and decide how fast or slow they will progress.

In Braking and Acceleration, lowering the volume on feelings of distress is the central requirement. Any activity that achieves this can likely be modified to assist clients. This may include humor, breathing, talking about a favorite activity or person, imagining safety, and holding a transitional object, among other activities. Some of these methods have already been covered in this text and some new ones will be added in subsequent sections.

After trauma processing begins, we need to have a series of approaches to suggest when things get too hot. Sometimes nothing seems to work and we must drop all "techniques" and simply provide a safe and reassuring holding environment for the client's grief and discomfort. Alternatively, we might suggest an imagined barrier between the person and their traumatic memories or cycle through any or all of the approaches we have utilized successfully in the past.

The following three exercises are Braking and Acceleration tools that have been used successfully for many years. Other excellent suggestions can be found in Rothschild (2000).

Layering (RE – CR)
(Baranowsky, 1997)

Time required: One or more sessions.
Materials required: Paper and pencil for therapist.
Indications for use: Use when the primary need is to enhance physical, cognitive, and emotional coping skills in the Trauma Memory Processing stage of trauma recovery.
Counterindications: Actively dissociating or dissociates during exercise; respiratory ailments.

This approach draws on techniques that the client will have already begun to utilize through the earlier stages of trauma therapy. Deep breathing is a central component to this approach. The client needs to be familiar with and competent in the use of a deep breathing method prior to utilizing Layering. It is possible to teach deep breathing in the same session prior to introducing the Layering approach. The individual is informed of the entire procedure prior to commencing. This exercise can be used when clients arrive for sessions with a heightened sense of distress over a recent or current event that is related to, but not necessarily a direct memory of, the traumatic event. Over time, after clients become skilled at Layering, they can use this approach on their own as a mastery technique for managing feelings of distress. A Layering – Charting form is also included for the clinician's use. *Note:* For clients who are unable to utilize deep breathing, this can be substituted with Comfort in One Part, especially when using the exercise of focusing on Comfort in the Palms of the Hands described in that exercise.

Delivery of Approach

This exercise is begun with the Ericksonian approach commonly referred to as the YES SET (I. Bilash, personal communication, February 19, 1997).

To establish the YES SET, recognize the individual's distress, then state the obvious to achieve consent.
A good statement to begin with is: "I see you are feeling upset about X (the identified trauma or concern). I know you want to be able to handle this in the best way possible."

You will generally get consent or a yes in response to this statement.

The next statement is "I would like us to work to together to your goal, is that okay?"
Again, you will likely receive a yes. Now we move toward a description of the exercise and again await consent.

You can start your description of Layering as follows:

"We have worked on deep breathing before. Because it has helped you in the past, we can use this approach to give you a sense of mastery over your own feeling of discomfort related to X. In this exercise, we speak about the disturbing event and then work on the deep breathing. In this way, you will be able to take breaks from telling your story, thus keeping the feelings from overwhelming you while still having the opportunity to speak about what has occurred."

1. Identify the source of discomfort or disturbing memory. Rate it on a 1-to-10 SUDs scale.
2. Remind the client of the deep breathing approach. Have them practice with three to five deep inhalations and exhalations (or focus on Comfort in One Part). Encourage them to follow the directions as described in the deep breathing exercise found in this text.
3. Tell them about Layering and how the exercise will progress.
4. Ask them to begin by telling you what has occurred or what keeps their memory disturbing. Request that they keep their expression as descriptive and succinct as possible to begin with. Tell them that you may interrupt them when you notice their breathing begin to change.
5. As they begin describing the event, keep an eye on their breathing, ask them to stop their description when you recognize a noteworthy change in their breathing (it will become shallow and rapid or labored).

6. Now have them focus inwardly and begin five deep inhalations and exhalations in the prescribed manner. After the fifth exhalation, have the individual focus outwardly again. Take a SUDs rating based on how they feel now. If the SUDs is higher than 5, ask them to take five more deep breaths; if it is 5 or lower, ask them to tell you more about the event that is causing them discomfort.
7. Follow steps 4 through 6 until the SUDs rating has been consistently reduced to below 5 while the client describes the entire event.

USING THE TOOLS
Layering
(Baranowsky, 1997)

A Mastery Approach to Disturbing Physical and Emotional Sensations

Target Event	SUDs
Emotional Reaction	
Thought – What is it that makes this event so upsetting?	
Outcome – What happened?	
DEEP BREATHING (5 times) (or Comfort in One Part)	
Target Event (Further description)	
DEEP BREATHING (5 times)	
Cognition (What thoughts go along with this experience?)	
DEEP BREATHING (5 times)	
Emotion (What feelings do you have about this event?)	
DEEP BREATHING (5 times)	
Body Sensation (What feelings of discomfort do you have in your body?)	
DEEP BREATHING (5 times)	
Emotion (What feelings do you have about this event?)	
DEEP BREATHING (5 times)	
Emotion (What feelings do you have about this event?)	

Alternatives (Refer to Comfort in One Part or Positive Self-Talk / Thought Replacement in this book.)
Continue with this process until SUDSs rating is below 5 for the identified event prior to ending the exercise. If this is not achieved, then end with a Safety and Stabilization Grounding exercise for closure.

Note: This page may be reproduced by the purchaser for clinical use.

From: Anna B. Baranowsky, J. Eric Gentry, & D. Franklin Schultz, *Trauma Practice: Tools for Stabilization and Recovery.* © 2011 Hogrefe Publishing

Comfort in One Part (RE)

Time required: 10 minutes.
Materials required: None.
Indications for use: Use when the primary need is to enhance physical coping skills in the Trauma Memory Processing stage of trauma recovery.
Counterindications: None.

This exercise assists the individual in using bodily-felt sensations to retrain the body to a new state of comfort or relaxation. After they have achieved this state they are now able to retain calmness, even if it is in only one small part, while facing difficult memories. In this way, they are now able to reassure and soothe themselves through the maintenance of Comfort in One Part while bravely forging ahead in resolution of past experiences.

Delivery of Approach

This approach was initially introduced in Erickson's work (Erickson & Rossi, 1989) and later revisited by Dolan (1991, p. 26). The individual is taught to deeply and completely relax one part of their body (this can be a part of their choosing). The process can be achieved through inductions described earlier in this text (Anchoring, Deep Breathing, or Safe-Place Imagery). After the individual is deeply relaxed they are instructed to select a part of their body that is prepared to completely release all tension and relax. They are encouraged to let this part feel a complete sense of ease, calmness, and a soft and deep contentment. Allow them time to fully feel that sense of comfort and to let it soak into that body part. After they give you a cue (lifted finger) that they have fully enjoyed this experience, ask them to return their attention slowly to the room in which they are seated.

The client has now prepared themself to retain Comfort in One Part while agreeing to proceed with traumatic memory processing. During the processing or telling of the story, they are instructed to monitor the body part that retains comfort. The body part becoming aroused out of comfort is the signal to take a break and find comfort again.

Comfort in the Palms of the Hands. A good approach to begin with is to have the individual focus on the center of the palms of their hands. Instruct the client to imagine warm sun beaming into the center of the palms of their upturned hands. Encourage sensory feelings of warmth and relaxation soothing and smoothing out the sensation of release in the center of the palms of the hands. Allow the individual to imagine the warmth spreading and easing any discomforts they may have.

A Time-Line Approach (RE – CR)
(Gentry, personal communication, 2002)

Time required: 20–30 minutes.
Materials required: Paper and pencil.
Indications for use: Use when the primary need is to enhance physical, cognitive, and emotional coping skills in the Trauma Memory Processing stage of trauma recovery.
Counterindications: Actively dissociating or dissociates during exercise.

What follows is an approach that incorporates much that is useful of the techniques for Braking and Acceleration, Self-Soothing, Systematic Desensitization, Looped Tape Scripting (presented shortly), Cognitive Restructuring, and Reciprocal Inhibition. Recall from a cognitive-behavioral perspective that Reciprocal Inhibition (relaxation with exposure to memories of a traumatic event) and Cognitive Restructuring helps mitigate the negative sequelae of traumatic stress. Whereas there are a number of available techniques with more or less research to support them to address posttraumatic stress difficulties, the manner in which you accomplish Reciprocal Inhibition and Cognitive Restructuring is limited only by your creativity.

Delivery of Approach

This approach is grounded in the notion of Reciprocal Inhibition and Cognitive Restructuring with a self-controlled start – stop element. It may be done in a group setting or it may be done in individual therapy. This technique is, of course, done after safety and stabilization has been successfully attained and the client has adequate skills for self-soothing. Self-soothing skills should include the ability to relax using exercises, self talk, breathing, etc. In this exercise, the therapist will act as a witness and monitor the distress level of the client. In a group setting, a partner can fill this role.

Steps:
1. Identify the specific traumatic event to be processed.
2. Have the client take an 8.5" × 11" sheet of paper, turn it the long way and draw a timeline in the middle like the following:

[_____]
Beginning   End

3. Have the client relax completely and ask them to view the event from a distance. Without actually fully entering the memory, have them start at the beginning of the event and separate it into time segments. This is similar to the Trigger List exercise earlier. They may separate it into as many segments as they like.
4. Then have them draw a line up from the timeline on their paper to indicate each segment in the order it occurs and label it with a word to help remind them of which segment it is.
5. Have them make the height of each line indicate the SUDs level (from 1 to 10) associated with each segment.

Now have them relax. They have just created a symbolic representation of the traumatic event. They may begin to process this at any time they have relaxed and their SUDs level is at 0 or 1, or they may wish to leave it and come back later. When they choose to begin, proceed as follows:

Steps:
1. Starting at the beginning, have them narrate the events of the first segment of the timeline.
2. Monitor their SUDs level. If it begins to rise too quickly and the client feels overwhelmed, they may wish to break that segment into smaller segments. If SUDs levels rise and the client does not feel overwhelmed, have them continue to narrate that segment and that segment only.
3. Stop at the end of the segment.
4. Have them begin self-soothing exercises. As they relax, ask them to discuss whatever comes to mind with you.
5. When their SUDs level has reached 0 or 1, they may choose to continue, or may choose to wait. If they choose to wait, they may leave the representation of the event with you, explaining to them that you are capable of keeping it until they are ready to finish. They do not have to take the event home with them. If they choose to proceed, repeat steps 1 through 5 of the second set of steps for the next segment on the timeline.

By the time they have finished, they will have worked their way completely through a traumatic memory, creating a narrative of the event that includes insights gained from the process. And they have done so without being overwhelmed by emotion. To further facilitate the processing of the event, it would be helpful for you to then retell the story back to them as accurately as possible. The client should continuously practice self-soothing exercises while this is being done. In a group setting this can be accomplished by having it read to the group by their partner.

Biofeedback (R – RE – CR)

Time required: Varies.
Materials required: Varies.
Indications for use: Use when the primary need is to enhance physical coping skills in the

Delivery of Approach

Biofeedback is simply any technique that provides the client with regular and ongoing feedback on one or more of their physiological responses to imaginal and/or *in vivo* stimuli. This can be as simple as monitoring (or helping the client to self-monitor) respiration rate to as

Trauma Memory Processing stage of trauma recovery.
Counterindications: Actively dissociating or dissociates during exercise.

sophisticated as watching positron emission tomography (PET) scans. Most commonly used are computer-aided monitoring of blood pressure, respiration, heart rate, skin temperature, and skin electrical conductivity (electrogalvanic skin response [EGR]). These monitoring techniques are used in conjunction with relaxation strategies to help the client "memorize" thoughts and behaviors that produce visible lowering of anxiety responses (e.g., elevation of skin temperature in the hands, lowered heart rate, lowered respiration, lowered EGR). The EmWave® product available at http://www.heartmath.com is an excellent example of a biofeedback system that is well researched, easy to operate, and efficient in providing a feedback system for client use. Clinicians can set up the system in their office and train the individual on the system and then use the biofeedback to monitor change while initiating an exposure exercise. This will enable the client to focus on their trauma memory while monitoring their heart rate and breathing. They can stop trauma exposure to relax, thereby improving the feedback from the system, and then resume the exposure exercise.

This technique has specific application in trauma treatment by allowing the client to have ongoing awareness of their arousal level while they are accessing and confronting trauma memories. This feedback stimulates the client to activate a relaxation response, therefore invoking reciprocal inhibition while renegotiating and resolving trauma memories.

2. Cognition

The following section describes a number of techniques that address the cognitive coping skills of traumatized individuals. Trauma survivors are likely to present with any number of cognitive distortions about themselves and the world in which they live, created as a way to make sense of their world and be safe. These distortions often result in significantly problematic behaviors. The recovery of clients from traumatic events includes not only processing the events themselves, but also identifying and restructuring the beliefs that have proven to be less than useful in managing their lives. It is also important to remember that trauma and particularly stress have a negative impact on one's ability to think, for reasons discussed earlier. Clients who are actively dissociating and/or are clearly experiencing ongoing, unmanaged stress in their lives may have difficulty performing these techniques because they will have difficulty thinking clearly. Stress issues and dissociation should be addressed first to achieve optimum outcome.

Downward Arrow Technique (RE – CR)

Time required: 5–30 minutes.
Materials required: None
Indications for use: Use when the primary need is to enhance cognitive coping skills in the Trauma Memory Processing stage of trauma recovery.
Counterindications: Client appears confused, stressed, and/or actively dissociating, or dissociates during exercise.

This approach, initially introduced by Burns (1980), is particularly useful when working with intrusive thoughts that inhibit recovery. The following illustration exhibits how to apply this approach when intrusive negative thoughts overwhelm individuals. In many cases, the greatest source of distress is linked to the notion that one must not have negative or intrusive thoughts, which leaves the individual with an additional internal battle. It is necessary to shift the battle to a challenge of beliefs to lessen the impact of the intrusive material.

Delivery of Approach

Example:
Polly is a 36-year-old woman who has negative intrusive thoughts related to an experience of childhood sexual abuse when she was 6 years old.

Automatic thoughts related to a traumatic or disturbing event: What happened to me is my fault.
Challenging statement: And if that were true, what would it mean? (This statement or some variation is repeated until fundamental or core beliefs are revealed.)
Automatic thoughts: I was a very bad girl.
Challenging statement: And if you were a "bad girl," what makes that thought upsetting to you?
Automatic thoughts: Everyone would know I am dirty and disgusting.
Challenging statement: If you were "dirty and disgusting," what then? What is the meaning of this to you?
Automatic thoughts: People would hate me and I need to feel loved.

We continue to process downward until the individual feels some lightening of the impact of their negative thought or hits a core belief at the source of their grief.

Core Belief: I am not loveable.

Once the client has revealed their core beliefs you can now focus on the following:

Do you wish to keep this belief?
The client will likely say "no" or "I don't know how to change." As this point, explain the following: it is possible to "install" a positive alternative to the internal core belief.

Identify the opposite to the core belief:
(You can aid the client in identifying this. Remember, the goal is to find the opposite, not to ensure that the client believes the opposite in this moment. That will come in time.)
I am loveable. I am good enough.

Initially, we can expect that the opposite to the core belief will lead the client to feel some discomfort, but just as it is true that exposure to disturbing events combined with relaxation leads to extinction of discomfort, it is also true that exposure to the positive combined with relaxation can lead to a calm, comfortable, and integrated response.

The goal now becomes exposure to the new positive alternative belief. Instruct your client to listen or repeat the new positive alternative until the SUDs rating when reflecting on this new belief is a 5 or lower.

Cognitive Continuum (CR)

Time required: 5–30 minutes.
Materials required: None.
Indications for use: Use when the primary need is to enhance cognitive coping skills in the Trauma Memory Processing stage of trauma recovery.
Counterindications: Client clearly confused, unmanaged stress, actively dissociating, or dissociates during exercise.

Baer (2001, p. 102) recommends the use of a Cognitive Continuum to further challenge negative beliefs about oneself. This is an especially useful technique when an individual arrives at a rigidly held negative belief that has a traumatic basis. For example, Polly, the same woman discussed above who had experiences of early childhood sexual abuse, arrives at the negative conclusion that she is "extremely bad" and "despised by others" for her involvement in the abuse.

This approach is also useful when dealing with clients who make pronouncements of themselves that are harsh generalizations and not based on reality.

For example, a client declares that she is a "terrible mother." One would think that a blanket statement like this might be based on something quite significant, but when the woman is questioned she admits to the following:
1. She makes meals for her children daily.
2. She takes them to school and picks them up.

3. She never hits them and rarely raises her voice.
4. She reads to them at bedtime.
5. She finds interesting activities for them to engage in after school and during weekends.
6. She regularly brings them to socialize with family and friends.

So what did this woman do? *She forgot to pack her child's lunch and the teacher called her about it.*

When she was speaking about the forgotten lunch it was with such utter self-contempt that there was absolutely no space for all the good things that she does every day in parenting her children.

Delivery of Approach

This is an exercise to aid people to gain perspective on their behaviors and better respond to their own normal shortcomings.

We begin to catalogue a range of truly "bad" things that occur daily in our society. Start with the following question: What things might go on a list of truly bad behaviors?

Example:
You will see checkmarks to the right of the item signifying, to perception of best to worst, the item ranked for the individual (we are not endorsing a ranking, only recognizing a given client's ranking):

	0 (best)	50 (neutral or ok)	100 (worst)
1. Being a serial killer			✗
2. Molesting a child			✗
3. Hitting a pedestrian with a car			✗
4. Punching a spouse			✗
5. Drinking and driving			✗

We also need to develop a list of good or neutral behaviors. What kinds of things might go on a list of good or neutral behaviors?

Example:
You will see checkmarks to the right of the item signifying to perception of best to worst the item ranked for the individual (we are not endorsing a ranking only recognizing a given client's ranking)

	0 (best)	50 (neutral or ok)	100 (worst)
1. Feeding the cat		✗	
2. Buying a loved one a gift for no reason		✗	
3. Sharing a laugh with a friend	✗		
4. Discovering a cure for cancer	✗		

Now we ask the client to rate all these items from 0 to 100 using the following rating scale below:
0 = best ever behavior
50 = neutral or okay behavior
100 = worst or most despicable behavior

After all the items are listed and rated, the client is then asked to add their own item. In our example, the client adds "I forgot to pack my child's lunch" to the list. Suddenly her conclusion that "I am a terrible mother" changed to "I guess I just got busy that morning and forgot. It was a good thing that the teacher called so she should make sure my child got her lunch."

USING THE TOOLS
Cognitive Continuum

Negative Declaration (write out the negative statement or belief below):
_____
_____

List your good qualities related to this situation:
_____
_____

Give examples of truly bad behaviors or occurrences:

          0 (best)   50 (neutral or ok)   100 (worst)

_____
_____
_____
_____

Give examples of good or neutral behaviors:

          0 (best)   50 (neutral or ok)   100 (worst)

_____
_____
_____
_____

Now add and rate the negative declaration:

          0 (best)   50 (neutral or ok)   100 (worst)

_____
_____
_____
_____

Note: This page may be reproduced by the purchaser for clinical use.

From: Anna B. Baranowsky, J. Eric Gentry, & D. Franklin Schultz, *Trauma Practice: Tools for Stabilization and Recovery.* © 2011 Hogrefe Publishing

Calculating True Danger (CR)

Time required: 10–30 minutes.
Materials required: Paper and pencil.
Indications for use: Use when the primary need is to enhance cognitive coping skills in the Trauma Memory Processing stage of trauma recovery.
Counterindications: Client clearly confused, unmanaged stress, actively dissociating, or dissociates during exercise.

Baer (2001, p. 102) suggests another useful technique for challenging negative cognitive beliefs. This is useful when feelings of safety are compromised – a common occurrence among trauma survivors. Use this exercise only when you are assured that true probability of an event will be much less likely than perceived by the client. For example, Sheldon believes that if he takes a much-needed vacation to a destination where he must fly, his flight will certainly crash and he will die.

This is a good example to work with because we know that globally more than 3 million people fly daily on commercial aircraft. In 1998, the world's airlines carried approximately 1.3 billion passengers on 18 million flights worldwide while suffering only 10 fatal accidents. Risk of being involved in a commercial aircraft accident resulted in one fatality per 3 million passengers that year. To put this in perspective, you would have to fly once every day for more than 8200 years to accumulate 3 million flights. Flying by commercial airliner is believed to be 22 times safer than driving your own car.

In cases where there is a real imminent and personal danger, we would not use this exercise of calculating true danger.

Delivery of Approach

Example:
First, Sheldon is given the opportunity to estimate the probability that his flight will crash (he believes the probability of this event is 25%). The next step is for Sheldon to work with the therapist to identity each step required for the feared outcome to occur. After all events leading up to "dying in a plane crash" are identified, each are again given a rating based on an assumed "chance of this event occurring." Then a "cumulative chance of all events" is calculated (see Table 5). Given our example of Sheldon's fear of dying in a plane crash, let us identify events and calculate the true probability of danger. Despite Sheldon's deep fear, he assesses the following events and still arrives at a very low percentage of probability using the exercise above. In this case, Sheldon's own estimate produces a chance of danger at the remarkably low 0.0000001%. This is a vast contrast from his pre-existing perceived fear of dying in a plane crash of 25% probability. This is a good example of how we can assist our clients in challenging their own notions of actual versus perceived fears.

Table 5. Calculating the true probability of danger

Event	Chance of this event occurring	Cumulative chance of all events
1. Sheldon must select a flight with some mechanical or other problem that will lead to a crash.	1 / 1000	1 / 1000
2. The error or problem will not be noticed before takeoff	1 / 10	1 / 10,000
3. The pilot, staff, or passengers will not be able to correct the problem while in air	1 / 10	1 / 100,000
4. There will be a crash landing	1 / 10	1 / 1,000,000
5. Sheldon will not survive the crash	1 / 10	1 / 10,000,000
Adapted from Baer, 2001, p. 102		

Looped Tape Scripting (RE – CR)

Time required: 10–60 minutes.
Materials required: Paper and pencil.
Indications for use: Use when the primary need is to enhance cognitive and emotional coping skills in the Trauma Memory Processing stage of trauma recovery.
Counterindications: Client clearly confused, unmanaged stress, actively dissociating, or dissociates during exercise.

This is a particularly challenging exercise. However, if we have built in all of the precautions with our clients as suggested in this text, they will likely be prepared to proceed with some reassurances. Looped Tape Scripting is an approach based on exposure therapy and habituation to the feared memory or thoughts. This requires the clinician to be skilled in handling disturbing clinical material and be able to stay calmly present for the client during the entire session.

Habituation occurs over time, when we are exposed to situations, memories, thoughts, or occurrences that may have caused distress or discomfort initially but over time become commonplace and no longer create the same level of distress. This requires practice and tolerance for initial discomfort. Research consistently shows improvement over time through the use of this exposure technique. Most of us can understand the notion of habituation when we recall times where we were initially annoyed or disturbed by something that over time we completely forgot about (i.e., a fear of the dark; a noise in our car; the sound of airplanes or traffic when we move into a new apartment; a distracting open-concept work environment, etc.). Remarkably, it also works the same way with much more disturbing material.

Note: Looped Tape Scripting can also be used to install positive cognitive or new core beliefs, such as those identified in the Downward Arrow technique.

Delivery of Approach

In this exercise, the individual is asked to identify a memory or a perceived fear or threat that they are prepared to work on with the goal of resolution at this time. Recall the Trigger List developed earlier in this book during Braking and Acceleration Part I. The Trigger List can provide the basis for selecting an event. When an event is selected, ask the individual to give it a SUDs rating from 1 to 10.

Now the individual is requested to write out the worst parts of the event or anticipated fear in great detail. Using this document, the individual is now encouraged to speak into a tape recorder or video camera. The entire script is read repeatedly until 30 minutes of recording is completed. The recorded document is now watched or listened to during the clinical session at least once. Their homework is to watch or listen to the script for an hour each day until the tape no longer results in a heightened SUDs rating. In this way, the individual achieves habituation to the feared past event.

The time required for habituation is different for each individual and clinicians need to have great tolerance for individual differences in processing time.

USING THE TOOLS
Looped Tape Scripting – Installing the Positive

Memory or Fear   SUDs = _____

_____

_____

_____

An alternative method is to itemize positive self-statements that the client is not yet comfortable with and use this list to work with the exposure method outlined in the Delivery of Approach for Looped Tape Scripting.

Example:
The positive exposure list below provides a challenge to the individual to integrate new, more adaptive self-talk utilizing a Loop Tape Script exercise.
I am loveable.
I am wonderful.
I am brilliant.
I am successful.
I am exciting.
I am interesting.
I am fun.
I am attractive.

Read through the above list above once and then give it a SUDs rating.
SUDs = _____

Work with deep breathing, Comfort in One Part, or any other self-soothe exercise.

Read through the list again working with the self-soothe method of choice.

Rate the SUDs again:
SUDs = _____

Continue with the exercise above until the SUDs rating is 5 or below.

Note: This page may be reproduced by the purchaser for clinical use.

From: Anna B. Baranowsky, J. Eric Gentry, & D. Franklin Schultz, *Trauma Practice: Tools for Stabilization and Recovery.* © 2011 Hogrefe Publishing

Cognitive Processing Therapy (RE – CR)

Time required: One to several sessions.
Materials required: Paper and pencil.
Indications for use: Use when the primary need is to enhance cognitive coping skills in the Trauma Memory Processing stage of trauma recovery.
Counterindications: Client clearly confused, unmanaged stress, actively dissociating, or dissociates during exercise.

Delivery of Approach

This approach was developed expressly to treat rape victims and incorporates both techniques of Cognitive Therapy and Exposure Therapy. In using the techniques of Cognitive Therapy, the clinician works to assist the survivor in confronting and restructuring the problematic cognitions that result from their traumatic experiences, especially self-blame (Resick & Schnicke, 1992, 1993). Building upon the work of McCann and Pearlman (1990), this approach also asks the survivor to address overgeneralized and often distorted beliefs about trust, power/control, self-esteem, and intimacy. Exposure Therapy techniques are utilized by asking the client to write a detailed account of their traumatic experience(s) and reading it back to the therapist as well as other willing witnesses. This intervention predicts the loosening of affect, which, in turn, often helps the survivor navigate through "stuck points" that they have heretofore been unable to either recall and/or move through.

USING THE TOOLS
Cognitive Processing Therapy

Follow the steps below:

1. Identify the unresolved memory, concern, or situation:
   _____
   _____

2. For 1 minute, remain in quiet reflection, letting your thoughts run with no judgment on the content. This should be a timed minute ending when a buzzer goes off.
   _____
   _____

3. Now take as much time as needed to write out the details of your thoughts during your 1-minute reflection, leaving out nothing (add paper if needed).
   _____
   _____
   _____
   _____
   _____
   _____
   _____
   _____
   _____
   _____
   _____

4. Repeat steps 2–3 until the SUDs ratings are 5 or less.
   _____
   _____

Note: This page may be reproduced by the purchaser for clinical use.

From: Anna B. Baranowsky, J. Eric Gentry, & D. Franklin Schultz, *Trauma Practice: Tools for Stabilization and Recovery.* © 2011 Hogrefe Publishing

A Story-Book Approach (RE – CR)
(Gentry, personal communication, 2002)

Time required: 10–30 minutes.
Materials required: Paper, colored markers.
Indications for use: Use when the primary need is to enhance cognitive coping skills in the Trauma Memory Processing stage of trauma recovery.
Counterindications: Client clearly confused, unmanaged stress, actively dissociating, or dissociates during exercise.

Delivery of Approach
Another technique that utilizes reciprocal inhibition and cognitive restructuring is the Story-Book Approach. Have your client identify the event on which they would like to work. Divide the event into at least four segments from beginning to end, timewise. (This may be used in conjunction with the timeline created in the previous technique or done separately.) Then take a sheet of paper and draw each segment. This can be done in comic-strip format or any other style the client chooses. Have the client practice continuous self-soothing while they complete the drawing and monitor their reactions to remind them. When the drawing is finished, have them tell the narrative using the pictures as a guide. Then retell the story back to them as accurately as possible. In a group setting, the drawing can be shown to the group and the narrative told by a partner.

A Written Narrative Approach (RE – CR)
(Gentry, personal communication, 2002)

Time required: 10–30 minutes.
Materials required: Paper and pencil.
Indications for use: Use when the primary need is to enhance cognitive coping skills in the Trauma Memory Processing stage of trauma recovery.
Counterindications: Client clearly confused, unmanaged stress, actively dissociating, or dissociates during exercise.

Delivery of Approach

Here is another technique that utilizes reciprocal inhibition and cognitive restructuring. Have your client write out the context of what occurred in as much detail as they care to include. As before, have them self-soothe as they are writing their story. After they have written about what happened, have them write down what they think they have lost because of the events. Finally, have them write what they think they might have gained as a result of what happened. They may then read it to you and/or have it read back to them.

3. Behavior

The most obvious indicator of successful treatment for trauma is the ability to translate this new learning into behavior. Is the client more relaxed? Are they better able to interact with others socially? Have they decreased self-defeating behaviors and less-than-useful self-soothing behaviors? Our clients have often spent a lifetime performing behaviors used to adapt to difficult circumstances and do not always have a repertoire of more useful behaviors. Also, performing new behaviors is, in itself, anxiety provoking because individuals attempting the new behaviors cannot predict the outcome. The techniques that follow are useful in generating new behaviors and they provide practice for clients to become comfortable and less anxious before using new skills in their regular daily lives.

Behavior Change Rehearsal Exercise (RE – CR)

Time required: 10–30 minutes.
Materials required: None.
Indications for use: Use when the primary need is to enhance behavioral coping skills in the Trauma Memory Processing stage of trauma recovery.

This approach has been based on Grinder and Bandler's (1981) "New Behavior Generator" exercise. The technique is offered as a procedure to utilize the imagination as a process for eventually freeing actual behavior in more desirable directions. The steps that follow incorporate several techniques introduced earlier (i.e., YES SET, Safety Anchor, or Visualization to a Safe Place). This technique can be used in Stress Inoculation Training as the "imaginary rehearsal" component that is integral to that approach.

Counterindications: Client clearly confused, unmanaged stress, actively dissociating, or dissociates during exercise.

Delivery of Approach

1. Identify the response or behavior the individual is dissatisfied with (e.g., cannot say no to overwork).
2. Identify all the payoffs to the current manner of handling this type of situation (e.g., everyone likes me; no one laughs at me).
3. Identify the disadvantages to maintaining the current behavior (e.g., I am exhausted; I feel others take advantage of me).
4. Which weighs more or has greater appeal: the payoffs for staying the same or the disadvantages? Do you want to stay the same or is it too painful to stay the same?
5. What alternative positive behavior could you substitute for the current behaviors?
6. Set up an "ideomotor" signal for yes and no (e.g., yes = thumbs-up; no = thumbs-down).
7. Determine which type of grounding to relaxation or safety you wish to use for this exercise (e.g., Anchoring Safety, Safe-Place Visualization, Progressive Relaxation, Autogenics). Prepare the individual for this "induction."
8. Once grounded in safety, ask the individual to do the following:
   a. Imagine that part of you remains in safety while another part of you acts as an observer and steps away from safety.
   b. Recall a past experience that left you feeling dissatisfied with your behavior.
   c. Once you can recall this memory, show me a thumbs-up to let me know you have the memory. Say "good" when you see thumbs-up.
   d. Imagine you are going to watch a videotape of this memory. You have the controls to start or stop the tape as you wish.
   e. Rewind the experience to just before the unpleasantness. Show me a thumbs-up when you are at the beginning of the tape.
   f. Play it all the way through to the end. Watch yourself behave in the manner that you wish to change. Remember you are an observer still grounded in safety.
   g. Now recall what new behavior you would like to replace for the old response. Give me a thumbs-up to let me know you have recalled the new behavior.
   h. "Good." Now watch and listen to yourself as you replace the old response with the new desired behavior. Watch as you are able to handle this situation that in the past would have given you difficulty. Play the video all the way through to the end, watching the new behavior in the old situation.
   i. Show me a thumbs-up when you are done. "Good."
   j. Having observed this new behavior in the old situation, was it completely satisfactory to you? Show me a thumbs-up if you were completely satisfied and a thumbs-down if not.
9. If the answer to 8.j is yes, go through the script above imagining a future imagined scenario similar to the actual memory. Have the person imagine one that might have caused difficulty in the past but which they wish to practice this new behavior on.
10. If the answer to 8.j is no, replay the same script until they are satisfied with their rehearsed imagined behavior. After they are satisfied, follow step 9.

Skills Building Methods (CR)
(Foa, Keane, & Friedman, 2000)

Time required: 10–30 minutes.
Materials required: Paper and pencil.
Indications for use: Use when the primary need is to enhance cognitive coping skills in the Trauma Memory Processing stage of trauma recovery.

Delivery of Approach

This treatment method is designed and recommended for severely and/or retraumatized women (Foa, Keane, & Friedman, 2000). Cloitre (1998) offers the acronym STAIR (Skills Training in Affect and Interpersonal Regulation/Prolonged Exposure). In this model, clients are guided through skills training and development in three distinct areas:

1. identifying and labeling feeling states (especially feelings of threat);

Counterindications: Client clearly confused, unmanaged stress, actively dissociating, or dissociates during exercise.

2. tolerating distress and modulating negative affect; and
3. effectively negotiating difficult interpersonal relationships requiring assertiveness and self-regulation. See original text for details.

Imaginal and *In-Vivo* Exposure (RE)

Time required: One or more sessions.
Materials required: Varies.
Indications for use: Use when the primary need is to enhance behavioral and cognitive coping skills in the Trauma Memory Processing stage of trauma recovery.
Counterindications: Client unable to self-soothe, actively dissociating, or dissociates during exercise. This exercise requires a significant level of stability and self-soothing ability.

Imaginal and *in-vivo* (live) exposures rely on a willingness to expose oneself directly to the actual feared person, place, thing, or event. Following trauma, individuals may become extremely distressed when returning to the scene of the trauma or the item associated with the trauma. Unfortunately, it is possible and even common that traumatic memories and feared triggers become generalized to other areas of our lives. For example, if an individual is in a motor vehicle accident, they may fear entering a car and even fear trains, planes, boats, buses, and all other modes of transportation. Repeated exposure to anxiety-arousing stimuli without danger supposedly provides a corrective learning experience. It is our belief that simply exposing a client to the imagined or actual stimuli until resolution of anxiety occurs is potentially retraumatizing and we believe that relaxation is a necessary ingredient for resolution. A method such as Systematic Desensitization (presented shortly) titrates the exposure and provides the client with the experience of self-management of the anxiety. Nevertheless, Imaginal and *In Vivo* Exposures are sometimes quick and effective ways to address the traumatic event.

Delivery of Approach

1. Identify the feared person, place, thing, or event.
2. Provide a SUDs rating (1–10) that indicates the degree of distress associated with this stimulus.
3. Self-soothe until the current SUDs rating is below 3.
4. Either imagine the event or stimulus, or recreate the event or stimulus as closely as possible in real life (*in vivo*) to begin the exposure.

Exposure is continued until the SUDs rating drops below 50% of the original rating. Ratings are taken at regular intervals, approximately every 5–10 minutes. When the SUDs rating has dropped to below 50%, the therapist may assist the client in further lowering their current SUDs level to 3 or less. It is very important to allow the client time to discuss and process their experience of the exposure. When the individual demonstrates adequate self-soothing and self-rescue abilities, they may be given homework to complete the exposure task daily until SUDs levels continue to remain low during exposure.

Example:
It is best to start with a list of gradually increasing activities leading to the most feared thing. For someone who has been in a motor vehicle accident, you might generate a list similar to the one below:

		SUDs
1	Look at pictures of cars	5
2	Go to a parking lot	5
3	Touch a car's driver's seat	6
4	Sit in a passenger's seat	7
5	Sit in the driver's seat	8
6	Be a passenger in a moving vehicle	8
7	Be the driver in a moving vehicle	9

The goal for each of these gradual steps, whether imaginal or in vivo, is to expose the client to each step, lowering the SUDs to a manageable level before moving on to the next step and eventually extinguishing the list.

Stress Inoculation Training (RE – CR)

Time required: 8–14 sessions.
Materials required: Varies.
Indications for use: Use when the primary need is to enhance physical, cognitive, behavioral, and emotional coping skills in the Trauma Memory Processing stage of trauma recovery.
Counterindications: Actively dissociating or dissociates during exercise. Client must clearly have the ability to self-soothe and self-rescue.

This classical cognitive behavioral treatment approach to posttrauma recovery was developed and first presented by Meichenbaum in 1987 (Meichenbaum, 1994). There is considerable research expressing the efficacy of this approach. It is a well-accepted protocol in the field of trauma treatment. Stress Inoculation Training (SIT) teaches individuals coping skills and practice opportunities to enhance their mastery over disturbing stress responses. SIT generally consists of 8–14 sessions and can be applied in groups or among individuals.

This treatment approach is broken into three phases (the outline below is adapted from Meichenbaum, 1994):
- Phase 1: Conceptualization
- Phase 2: Skills Acquisition, Consolidation, and Rehearsal
- Phase 3: Application Training

Phase 1: Conceptualization
In this phase, the individual is informed of the treatment format and provided with psychoeducational training to better understand their symptoms and reactions. It is at this stage that the client works collaboratively with the therapist to identify positive coping strategies.

Phase 2: Skills Acquisition, Consolidation, and Rehearsal
In Phase 2, the clinician draws heavily from materials reviewed earlier in this text. This is the most complex and time-intensive part of the book. The core focus is cognitive, behavioral, and physiological (body) skills acquisition to moderate or manage feelings of stress, anxiety, fear, guilt, and anger. The individual is encouraged to make it their goal to change:
1. the stressful environment or situation whenever possible;
2. one's perception or "meaning" of the situation; or
3. emotional reactions evoked by the situation or recollections of disturbing occurrences.

Strategies for moderating or managing disturbing or stressful situations include:
1. Leave the situation.
2. Change the situation.
3. Accept the situation as it stands and achieve satisfaction or support in other areas of one's life.
4. Reframe the situation differently or develop new interpretations.

The goals and strategies listed above can be traversed through the utilization of many coping skills. It is during this phase that skills are taught and practiced. Skills covered include "direct-action and problem-focused coping and emotional-regulative palliative coping" (Meichenbaum, 1994, p. 394).

The coping skills taught in this section include relaxation exercises, positive self-talk or challenges to negative thinking, problem solving, distraction, etc. After skills are in place, individuals are taught to prepare, confront, and cope with disturbing events and feelings. When the event is over, they are encouraged to reflect on the effectiveness of the coping strategy and either reinforce or select another approach to stress management.

Phase 3: Application Training
Imaginary rehearsal, role-playing, and *in vivo* graduated exposure are applied in this phase. Relapse prevention through follow-up sessions is an integral part of SIT.

Delivery of Approach

The clinician can utilize the following steps to help the client complete the Stress Inoculation Exercise. After one or two trainings, the client will be able to initiate and complete this exercise without the aid of the clinician.

USING THE TOOLS
SIT Phase Oriented – Task Checklist

Phase 1: Conceptualization
1. This is the interview stage. Identify stressors and types of occurrences that are demanding for the individual.
2. Request narrative accounts of stressors and coping strategies. Identify available strengths and resources.
3. Deconstruct disturbing reactions as they relate to distressing incidents. Recognize automatic responses and coping resources. Assess the utility of each.
4. Clarify the difference between things you can change and those you cannot.
5. Begin the process of goal setting. Focus on achievable and specific tasks.
6. Achieve self-awareness of stress reactions and early warning signs (i.e., emotional, behavioral, physical, cognitive, relational). Using this awareness assist the individual to closely self-monitor.
7. Recognize coping deficits and identify for future training efforts.
8. Normalize stress response, reinforce the positive strengths utilized, and begin to bring meaning into one's perception of experiences.
9. Reassure that everyone responds to stress in a unique manner and there is no "right way."

Phase 2: Skills Acquisition and Rehearsal
1. Provide skills training that fit the individual or groups needs.
    e. Identify what works for the individual and how to reinforce this strength.
    f. Introduce problem-focused instrumental coping skills. Problems are broken into subcomponents that can be addressed individually. Appropriate skills are taught to manage a given problem.
    g. Begin solution-focused problem-solving activities that include recognizing desired change and rating alternative solutions. Introduce behavioral coping activities for in session and *in vivo* practice.
    h. Introduce emotionally focused palliative coping skills. These are essential when situations are beyond one's control and not likely to change. Helpful exercises include: relaxation, cognitive reframing, humor, and self-care.
    i. Encourage the use of social supports and introduce appropriate social skills development when required.
    j. A wide spectrum of skills development is required for long-term recovery or management of distress. Encourage a broad picture of coping resources.
2. Integrate a skills rehearsal component.
    a. Utilize imaginary and behavioral rehearsal activities to better prepare the individual for real-life use of new skills.
    b. Provide a demonstration (live or videotaped) of "coping modeling" (Meichenbaum, 1994, p. 397). The coping model displays both initial discomfort or distress and then resourceful coping strategies. Allow for discussion and rehearsal after the demonstration.
    c. Challenge negative self-defeating internal dialogue and reinforce positive adaptive self-talk.
    d. Make a commitment to future resourcefulness and resiliency efforts.
    e. Identify blocks to adaptive coping.

Phase 3: Application, Relapse Prevention, and Follow-Through
1. Application of adaptive coping skills:
    a. Utilize early stress warning signs to cue individual to access new coping skills in response to stress.
    b. Increase imagery exposure exercise to include more stressful and disturbing material.
    c. Integrate graded exposure techniques and in vivo exercises.
    d. Rehearse coping responses as a relapse prevention technique. Recognize trigger situations or occurrences and rehearse positive coping skills to stressful and automatic reactions.
    e. Involve the individual in recognizing the utility of any given exercise through direct questioning of where, how, and why skills will be used.
    f. Teach the individual to take "credit" for new skills development and utilization through "attribution retraining." Review successful and unsuccessful attempts to use new skills.

Note: These two pages may be reproduced by the purchaser for clinical use.

From: Anna B. Baranowsky, J. Eric Gentry, & D. Franklin Schultz, *Trauma Practice: Tools for Stabilization and Recovery.* © 2011 Hogrefe Publishing

2. Maintain new skills and then generalize to more situations.
    a. Spread out timing of sessions to include "booster and follow-up sessions" (Meichenbaum, 1994, p. 398).
    b. Involve family, friends, and other care providers in the ongoing success of the individual.
    c. Offer a coaching opportunity to the client so they can teach what they have learned. This is best attempted with group models.
    d. Make life changes where possible and encourage a sense of self-control through the establishment of "escape routes" where necessary.
    e. Reinforce a realistic attitude where there is recognition that life can be stressful at times and they will not handle every occurrence in an ideal manner. These times can simply be opportunities for learning and a chance to gain new skills. In this way, the individual can learn over time and not feel guilt or shame for perceived failures or setbacks.

Note: These two pages may be reproduced by the purchaser for clinical use.

From: Anna B. Baranowsky, J. Eric Gentry, & D. Franklin Schultz, *Trauma Practice: Tools for Stabilization and Recovery.* © 2011 Hogrefe Publishing

USING THE TOOLS
SIT Book Developer

The purpose of this exercise is to integrate teaching from this book by recognizing what approaches you can utilize to achieve each of the tasks required in this SIT Book Developer. Use the contents of this book as a resource and write the name of the approach you choose for each task required. See the SIT Checklist above for further details and explanations.

Note: There are additional tasks required during a full SIT found in the checklist.

Phase 1: Conceptualization

Identify your target group or individual:

_____

_____

Recognize automatic responses and how they are damaging or useful. Normalize stress responses and reinforce the positive.

_____

_____

Phase 2: Skills Acquisition and Rehearsal

Provide appropriate skills training for your individual or group.

_____

_____

Integrate a skills rehearsal component.

_____

_____

Phase 3: Application, Relapse Prevention, and Follow-Through

Encourage the use of specific coping skills.

_____

_____

Maintain new skills and generalize these to additional situations.

_____

_____

Note: This page may be reproduced by the purchaser for clinical use.

From: Anna B. Baranowsky, J. Eric Gentry, & D. Franklin Schultz, *Trauma Practice: Tools for Stabilization and Recovery.* © 2011 Hogrefe Publishing

Systematic Desensitization (RE)

Time required: One to several sessions.
Materials required: Paper and pencil for therapist.
Indications for use: Use when the primary need is to enhance behavioral coping skills in the Trauma Memory Processing stage of trauma recovery.
Counterindications: Actively dissociating or dissociates during exercise. Client must clearly have the ability to self-soothe and self-rescue.

Developed in 1969 by Joseph Wolpe, this technique is the basis for most behavioral treatments for anxiety and traumatic stress (Wolpe, 1969). Drawing upon the principles of reciprocal inhibition, Wolpe combined a hierarchy of negative associations with a triggering event or object with relaxation strategies. He theorized that, as the client was able to develop the *relaxation response* at each level of the hierarchy, they would then be able to accommodate a move to the next higher level of anxiety-producing stimuli. Systematic desensitization is said to be complete when the feelings of anxiety are *extinguished* with *in vivo* exposure to the original anxiety-producing situation or object.

Delivery of Approach

Example:
A client feels overwhelming anxiety when confronted with returning to work as a bank teller after a robbery.

1. Develop a hierarchy of real and imagined situations in which he would feel increasing levels of anxiety due to demands placed upon him in the work context.
   i. (SUDs = 10): serving customers from the same section where the robbery occurred;
   ii. (SUDs = 8): working at a bank station;
   iii. (SUDs = 6): entering the bank;
   iv. (SUDs = 4): parking at the bank;
   v. (SUDs = 2): driving past the bank.

2. Learn and master a set of self-soothing and anxiety-reduction behaviors and practices that the client can use to lessen arousal when confronted with anxiety-producing stimuli.
   a. Progressive Relaxation;
   b. Safe-Place Sisualization;
   c. Diaphragmatic Breathing;
   d. Positive Self-Talk.

3. The clinician then leads the client through an *imaginal exposure* of the hierarchy created above, beginning with the lowest SUDs level situation. After the client has demonstrated the ability to successfully lower his anxiety at the lowest level of exposure, the clinician guides him to the next level of anxiety-producing stimuli. This continues, often over several sessions, until the client has demonstrated the ability to remain calm when confronting the highest level of anxiety-producing stimuli.

4. The clinician then assists the client in seeking out *in vivo* situations that are similar to those above, during which he can practice relaxation while confronting situations that previously provoked anxiety.

4. Emotion/Relation

Survivors of traumatic events have often spent a lifetime avoiding their own emotions and appeasing others to ward off danger. Many times they lack not only emotional coping skills, but also interactive skills. The following techniques provide access to these skills to better enable clients to experience their own emotions without being overwhelmed and assist them with interacting with others without feeling or being overwhelmed.

Learning to Be Sad (CR)

Time required: One to several sessions.
Materials required: None.
Indications for use: When one needs to feel sad.
Counterindications: Inability to actively self-soothe.

This exercise is adapted from *A Language of the Heart Workbook*, by D. Franklin Schultz, PhD. It is especially useful when used in conjunction with the Creating a Nonanxious Presence technique. As in that technique, the first part is primarily psychoeducational, giving clients a different understanding of the meaning of sadness. It is not a replacement for trauma reduction techniques and, in fact, relates more to the everyday feelings we all must process. However, it is a very powerful technique that has the ability to elicit unprocessed and sometimes unremembered trauma and the feelings associated with it. Therefore, this technique should be done during sessions the first few times to insure the client has the self-soothing abilities to manage this unprocessed trauma and hold it for processing in session.

Delivery of Approach

Clients quickly recognize that their fear of sadness is one of the biggest blocks to their doing the work necessary for recovery. As they proceed in recovery, they begin reflecting on things they have managed to push outside of their consciousness for a long while. They actually begin to feel the sadness, dejection, disappointment, aloneness, or abandonment from these past experiences. And this is what they should do about that: – nothing! That, however, requires a bit of explaining. Dr. Schultz uses the following script when preparing clients for this technique.

USING THE TOOLS
Sadness Script

What we have been doing all along when we become sad is "something." We have been taught since we were children that it was not okay to be sad. We were called a "baby" and told to "grow up," or to "get over it," to "quit your crying," or (my favorite) "quit your crying or I'll give you something to cry about." We thus learned many ways to "stuff" our sadness. We deny, cover up, run, distract ourselves, get busy, drink, work, play, get angry, whatever it takes to stuff it. And the problem with stuffing our sadness is that it does not go away. It piles up. Soon the pile is so big we're afraid if we ever touch it, it will come roaring out and never stop. It will flood us, drown us, or leave us dead or dying. And so we stuff it.

The truth about sadness is that although it feels as if we will die or be overwhelmed by it, we actually will not. But we have to learn how to be sad – how to be sad without becoming reactive, doing something to "stuff" our sadness. Why, you ask, would someone want to do that? Because sadness is a normal, natural emotion. Sadness is about loss: loss of childhood, loss of innocence, loss of love, loss of relationship, loss of control, etc. Sadness has a unique ability to change a painful experience of loss into information about what is useful, important, and valuable or about what is not useful, not important, and not valuable in the choosing of our own behaviors. If we allow ourselves to feel our sadness all the way to the end of it (and there is a beginning, a middle, and an end), it will change the experience into information, and we will be better able to choose our own behaviors to avoid unneccesary harm to ourselves and others. In other words, sadness has the ability to change pain into wisdom. If we stop our sadness from running its course, we just manage to restuff it and never really learn the lessons.

We have this story that we tell ourselves. It is "our" story, about our life. It contains all of the experiences we have that we can think about that define us and tell us who we are. We tell others some of the story, but mostly it is a personal story. When we have painful experiences that we cannot think about because they are too painful and we have not grieved them, the experiences never have an opportunity to take their place in our stories. They never have an opportunity to inform us what is useful, important, and valuable or not useful, not important, and not valuable about what we experienced. Therefore, these experiences cannot provide us direction as we choose our own behaviors. When we allow ourselves to feel sadness all the way to the end, these experiences get to take their rightful place in our stories and we become wiser.

Consequently, the question is "how do you treat yourself when you are sad?" Is this difficult to answer? If you have children (even imaginary ones), you might ask " how do I treat my children when they are sad?" As it turns out, one of the best things we can do for our children is teach them how to be sad. Here is how: mostly by doing nothing! Of course, we make sure they are safe and loved, but then we should do nothing. We should just hold them. We should be kind and patient. We should *not* try to distract them from their sadness, tell them it is okay, tell them it is not important, give them an ice cream cone, or tell them to quit crying. We should just be with them. We might reassure them that they are loved. We might acknowledge their sadness and suggest that sometimes the world is a sad place. We might tell them we will be sad with them while they are sad because sometimes we are sad, too. Often, when this happens, children begin to open up about what they are feeling. They will tell you amazing little details about what they are worried about or what they have been sad about in the past. And this is what you should do: nothing. It is important to simply acknowledge this information. Do not try to fix it. Do not tell them it is nothing to worry about. Just acknowledge it. Your job is to be a witness. If you do not react to their sadness by shutting it down, when they are finished being sad they will usually get up and go play.

And this is how you learn to be sad with yourself: be kind and patient – with yourself. Do not listen to those words in the back of your head that say "grow up," "get over it," etc. Just be sad – without reacting to distract yourself. With permission, you may sob. Your tears may fall. Your nose may run. And this may last a day, a week, a month, or more. You may have weird thoughts and odd memories come up. If you are lucky enough to have a significant other who will hold you, ask them to not try to do anything to fix it. Just allow yourself to be sad. Eventually, you will come to the end of it. When you do, you will know it. You will feel strangely empty and light – as if a 5-ton weight had been lifted from your shoulders – and also sad. Oddly, you will also feel happy.

Note: These 3 pages may be reproduced by the purchaser for clinical use.

From: Anna B. Baranowsky, J. Eric Gentry, & D. Franklin Schultz, *Trauma Practice: Tools for Stabilization and Recovery.* © 2011 Hogrefe Publishing

Have you ever tried to sit on a beach ball in a swimming pool, trying to keep the beach ball completely under water? It takes lots of concentration and energy to struggle with the ball and it always seems to find its way back to the surface. Eventually you get tired of the game but the beach ball does not. Keeping your sadness from coming up into your consciousness requires tremendous concentration and energy; yet, like the beach ball, it seems to find its way to the surface much too often.

What if you let the air out of your beach ball of sadness? Then you could spend that energy doing something you really wanted to do – like feel good about yourself.

This does not mean you will never be sad again. Sadness is a constantly recurring emotion. In fact, a friend of mine thinks we may be sad as often as 10 or 15 times per day. We usually work harder, play harder, watch more television, drink more, or eat more to distract ourselves. However, when you learn to be sad when it is time to be sad, you then can get on with your life without carrying the burden of that huge bag of sadness and have more energy left over to do the things you really want to do. As you learn to be sad without reacting, you realize how often old sadness and fear from your past has dictated your behaviors.

This technique is somewhat unusual because you are being asked to allow yourself to feel things you have possibly pushed out of your awareness for a long time. If you experienced significant traumatic events in your childhood that are unresolved through personal work and/or therapy, this exercise has the potential of eliciting very strong emotions. Monitor yourself. Feeling completely overwhelmed is a good indication that you need to work on self-soothing skills. Talk with your therapist about how to more effectively accomplish that.

The Sadness Exercise:

For this exercise, you are asked to make an agreement with yourself to do nothing other than sit and be curious. You may stop any time you wish, especially if you are feeling overwhelmed. However, while you are doing the exercise, you should not do anything to avoid the feelings other than a self-soothing technique such as Creating a Nonanxious Presence. You should also make an agreement with yourself to not make any decisions about the information you think about. In other words, you may come to conclusions and think you need to go fix something right away. I suggest that you wait before you make any big decisions. When information comes up, just sit with it and let it process. Most of the things that arise will be old stuff. So just let it come up and witness it. Allow yourself to feel the perhaps long forgotten sadness associated with it. This exercise is not meant to affix blame or point fingers. It is a process by which you finally assimilate your past experiences and allow yourself to move forward.

To begin, find a comfortable place to sit where you will not be interrupted for an hour or two. This is very important. Schedule a specific amount of time to do this exercise. Make an agreement with yourself that you will do this exercise for exactly 1 hour or exactly 2 hours. You may even want to set a timer. Try to hold fairly exactly to this time frame. You will have plenty of time to do this exercise again. Do not imagine that you will get completely to the bottom of things in one sitting. Scheduling a specific amount of time and not exceeding it is a way for you to control what may, at first, seem overwhelming. This does not have to overwhelm you. It will, however, be emotional. Also, make sure to plan an additional hour after the exercise to relax. You will probably need a little additional relaxation time when you have finished.

Take some time to relax and breathe. Try to feel your connection to the earth. Give yourself permission to think about whatever comes up and feel whatever emotions arise with those thoughts. Make an agreement with yourself that your intent is to just witness what you have inside, not to "do" anything about it. Your goal is to begin to review your life and identify those experiences that left you feeling bad about yourself or sad. You may want to start by walking through your life year by year from earliest memories to more recent memories. Another possibility is to pick a movie you found especially difficult to watch because it made you emotional. Notice, especially, those areas where you might initially think you were just angry. Underneath the anger is, invariably, sadness. Make a space inside yourself for all of the emotions that might arise. Try not to reject *any* thought or emotion that comes up. Welcome these thoughts and emotions as information about how you came to think about yourself the way you do and how you came to behave to protect your heart.

Note: These 3 pages may be reproduced by the purchaser for clinical use.

This is not necessarily a pleasant experience at first. It sometimes may feel like a roller coaster out of control. Emotions will well up and come flooding out. Eventually, you may find yourself tearful or even sobbing. This is very important: *do not judge yourself.* If you are tearful, it does not mean that you are broken, bad, weak, stupid, or a baby. The stuff that is coming up is the stuff you have been hiding from your whole life. Be kind and gentle with yourself. Insist that you think of yourself with respect and dignity.

The best thing you can do when these emotions arise is keep your belly soft. Do a self-soothing technique such as Creating a Nonanxious Presence again and again. Breathe slowly and deeply and relax your belly. Keep your neocortex functioning. Remember where you are (in the here and now) at all times. Check that you are "safe." Allow yourself the right to be as sad as you need to be. Do not expect that you will "solve" all of your problems. Just relax and let whatever comes up come up.

The next step is very important. At the end of your allotted time, *stop* the exercise. Do not let it extend beyond your agreed-upon allotted time. You will always have time to come back and do it again. Take some time to fully ground yourself to the here and now. Take several slow, deep breaths. Open your eyes, if they are closed, and look around you. Relax your belly. Congratulate yourself for the courageous work you just accomplished. You will probably be somewhat to very tired. This is because you have just done some very difficult work. Take the next hour or so to relax. Treat yourself. Take a nap or a walk or try a nice bath or shower. Do whatever you like to just wind down. Do not, however, drink alcohol or caffeine or turn on the television. Allow yourself to decompress as slowly and naturally as possible.

Notice the language you are using with yourself. Did you immediately drop back into the old habit of scolding yourself for being weak? It is not true. *Relax your belly.* Remember, you gave yourself permission to do this. Some people report this to be a very difficult exercise because they are not used to letting go. Not only are they telling themselves that it is not okay, they are reminding themselves of what their friends and loved ones would say if they heard or saw them. This would be a very good time to work on your self-validation. This is your opportunity to let the air out of the beach ball. Your friends and loved ones may not understand that, so how can they have an opinion about what you are doing? You do not have to please them to accomplish this goal. In fact, take this as your first opportunity to be healthy for your own sake rather than someone else's.

Come back to this exercise as often as you like. You may find that you spontaneously begin to process sad information. Good! The object is to keep it flowing through you like water through a hose. You will find that once you give yourself permission to be sad, it will happen more often. However, now when it happens, it will not be nearly so painful and objectionable. We are sad every day – sometimes very sad, sometimes a little sad. Do not stuff it. Learn what it has to teach you.

There is only one follow-up question. Ask yourself, "What did I learn about what is important?" The insights you will get from doing the exercise will come for a significant amount of time after you have done it. You will have "aha!" experiences that seem to just pop into your mind that will help you understand significant pieces of your past and the pasts of those around you. Remain curious and keep your belly soft.

Note: These 3 pages may be reproduced by the purchaser for clinical use.

From: Anna B. Baranowsky, J. Eric Gentry, & D. Franklin Schultz, *Trauma Practice: Tools for Stabilization and Recovery.* © 2011 Hogrefe Publishing

Assertiveness Training (CR)

Time required: One to several sessions.
Materials required: None.
Indications for use: Use when the primary need is to enhance cognitive and emotional coping skills in the Trauma Memory Processing stage of trauma recovery.
Counterindications: Inability to actively self-soothe.

There are some basic principles to Assertiveness Training that are covered in most books. Primarily, individuals are assisted in achieving a sense of their rights and an ability to clearly state their wants, needs, and desires. Individuals are encouraged to move from "suffering in silence" to identifying unsatisfying situations or those that clearly violate our basic rights. With this knowledge, individuals are empowered to respond in a new and more personally gratifying manner to meet their own needs.

Delivery of Approach

Common tips include:
- Clearly state what you want, need, or prefer.
- Use "I" statements to declare negative emotions and dissatisfaction.
- Receive compliments simply with "thank you." Self-depreciating statements and other qualifiers are not required.
- Pose questions to tradition or authority when you are not satisfied with just going along.
- Share personal experiences, opinions, and feelings with confidence. Your viewpoint counts.
- Resolve frustrations and minor irritations before they escalate into major catastrophes and explosions of anger.
- Say no when you mean no. Saying yes will lead to feelings of resentment.
- Look at your own family of origin to identify where your submissive tendency developed.

There are many excellent resources on Assertiveness Training, including items found easily on the Internet through any search engine. Try http://www.mentalhelp.net for a starting point.

Practicing each of the tips above can assist clients in taking "assertiveness" from the clinician's office to their personal life.

Section 4
Reconnection

To be able to fill leisure intelligently is the last product of civilization.
Bertrand Russell

Reconnection

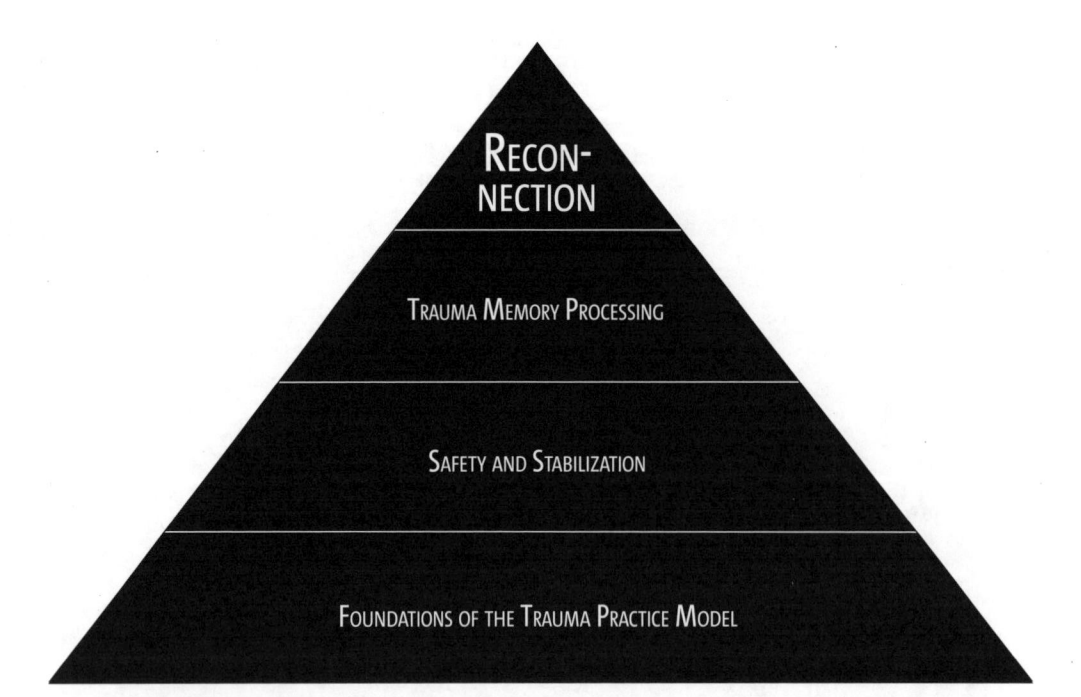

Trauma Memory Processing

Safety and Stabilization

Foundations of the Trauma Practice Model

1. Body
    Centering (CR)
2. Cognition
    Exploring Your Cognitive Map (CR)
    Victim Mythology (CR)
    Letter to Self (CR)
3. Behavior
    Self-Help and Self-Development (CR)
4. Emotion/Relation
    Memorials (CR)
    Connections with Others (RE – CR)

As the trauma is addressed in recovery, the emotional constriction and withdrawal that was useful in the past for safety begins to lift. The final stage of recovery involves redefining oneself in the context of meaningful relationships and engagement in life activities. Trauma survivors gain closure on their experiences when they are able to see things that happened to them with the knowledge that these events do not determine who they are. Trauma survivors are liberated by the conviction that, regardless of what else happens to them, they always have themselves. Many survivors are also sustained by an abiding faith in a higher power that they believe delivered them from oppressive terror. In many instances, survivors find a "mission" through which they can continue to heal and to grow. They may even end up helping others with similar histories of abuse and neglect. Successful resolution of the effects of trauma is a powerful testament to the indomitability of the human spirit. After Phase II of Trauma Practice is completed, personality that has been shaped through trauma must then be given the opportunity for new growth experiences that offer the hope of a widening circle of connections and the exploration of a broader range of interests.

1. Body

Many trauma survivors have spent a lifetime fighting the bodies they live in. They do not feel comfortable in their own skin. The behaviors they employed to keep themselves safe were often less than respectful to their bodies, or they just plain ignored their bodies. As they emerge from the emotional constriction of trauma, they begin the process of reconnection, including reconnection to their own bodies. Clients will find it useful to explore new ways to connect with themselves. Nutrition classes, exercise classes, Pilates, meditation, yoga, Tai Chi, Qigong, etc. are all useful and gentle ways to accomplish this. The following exercise is useful to help them "settle into their own skin" and begin the process of being aware of who they are.

Centering (CR)

Time required: As per Thich Nhat Hanh – forever.
Materials required: None.
Indications for use: Use when the primary need is to enhance physical, cognitive, behavioral, emotional, and relational coping skills in the Reconnection stage of trauma recovery.
Counterindications: Inability to actively self-soothe.

This exercise springs from the increasingly familiar work on "mindfulness" or reflection and acceptance. Or, as Jon Kabat-Zinn (1990) explains in his ground-breaking book *Full Catastrophe Living*, "Mindfulness is cultivated by assuming the stance of an impartial witness to your own experience" (p. 33). He goes on to state that, as we begin to pay attention to the internal dialogue, "it is common to discover and to be surprised by the fact that we are constantly generating judgments about our experience" (p. 33).

The next important piece of mindfulness is "acceptance." Without this we will make no progress because we cannot live peacefully within our own bodies if we are unable to gracefully accept its natural fragility along with its strength. If we are plagued with chronic headaches following a traumatic event, we will certainly be worse off if we grow angry and frustrated every time we have a headache. Our anger and frustration will fuel our headache, feeding it into a much worse bodily-felt experience.

Delivery of Approach

Thich Nhat Hanh (1990) explains a five-step process for centering that opens a dialogue between the individual and their internal bodily-felt experiences. He recommends that we allow ourselves to get to know and reflect on our internal processes, whether it is fear, pain, sadness, confusion, irritation, etc.

1. Just notice what comes up, leaving judgment aside.

2. Greet the internal experience (e.g., "Hello sadness. What is happening with you today? Why are you here?"). This is in contrast to the common response which may be "Hey, get out of here, sadness, you have no place inside of me! Who invited you?" In this way, we are no longer battling with ourselves. It becomes acceptable for us to feel whatever surfaces. The mindfulness is present and can moderate our internal experience of sadness – we are to just watch and let our attachment to judgment drop. Conscious breathing is an integral component to centering.

3. Coax an inner calmness just as you would soothe a young child who is feeling sadness or pain. You might say, "I am here, sadness, and I will not abandon you. I am breathing into my sadness with calm cooling breath." Being one with the feeling allows it the space and time to be nurtured, explored, expressed, and acknowledged, and provides the opportunity for respectful recovery.

4. Begin the process of releasing the feeling. You have faced the fearful emotion living in your body. It is now time to recognize that, as you add a calm mindfulness, the sadness begins to

transform. You have taught your body to feel at ease, even in the presence of deep sadness. You have sent a new message to your body: you are ready to remain present and care for yourself even when faced with disturbing internal messages. Make a conscious decision to soften the feeling even more, noticing that it can become a gentler expression. Imagine yourself smiling calmly at your feeling and letting it go with willingness to release.

5. Take a deeper look. Bring your mindfulness to the source of the discomfort. Even if it has fully dissipated, the body will have a memory of its existence. Ask, "What is this feeling about? Where did it come from? What internal or external causes form this experience?" With questions like this, we can better understand ourselves. With understanding, we can find the source of our internal distress. We can offer our own wise counsel, offering words of kindness and support, self-acceptance, and transformation.

This is a self-mastery exercise, one that can add to the richness of anyone's life.

2. Cognition

Even after resolving significant emotional reactions to trauma, clients are left with enduring patterns of how they think about themselves and the world. These are often very subtle patterns of thought that result in continued difficulties reconnecting to others. Just like a fish never thinks about the water he swims in, people never think about why they think the way they think – they just do it. It takes effort to identify these thoughts and then more effort to change them. The first step is to become consciously aware of them. The following techniques are useful to help clients become aware of some of these enduring patterns of thought.

Exploring Your Cognitive Map (CR)

Time required: A lifetime
Materials required: Paper and pencil.
Indications for use: When one needs to identify the situations and triggers that result in less than useful thought patterns.
Counterindications: Inability to actively self-soothe.

The following exercise is adapted from *A Language of the Heart: Therapy Stories that Heal*, by D. Franklin Schultz, PhD. At first, clients are not accustomed to thinking about how they think. Life just happens. As they explore their cognitive map, they will begin to realize they are different under different circumstances. They are mostly unconscious that they are different. However, as they become more conscious of their thoughts, they will eventually become more aware of themselves in the moment and begin to recognize the triggers or prompts for being different. After they become more conscious, they can become more intentional.

Delivery of Approach

What follows is a list of questions identified by others as significant in their development. The questions may help your clients begin to understand how they came to think about themselves and others and how they came to behave toward themselves and others. The questions cover different areas of early experience. The list is not exhaustive. For each question about an area of experience, your clients should ask themselves what impact these events had on their way of life. To what degree would they consider the impact to be positive or negative? How so? Specifically, have them consider the following questions when thinking about the impact:

1. What impact did these events have on your outlook, self-image, sense of safety, expectations, and relationships with others?

2. What are the beliefs about yourself that arose because of these events that you might question now?

3. What are the feelings the answers evoke and how do these relate to your current experience of the world?

4. What are the exact words you used to help you organize and understand the events to which they relate?

5. What are the exact triggers that remind you of these events?

As clients do this exercise, they should remember that the specific answer to each question is not as important as their own thoughts and emotional responses to the answer. Two people may have the same answer to the specific question and much different thoughts and emotional responses to their own meaning attached to the answer. They may notice a specific emotional charge to some of the questions. Have them pay attention to these and ask themselves whether situations in the here-and-now are similar to past events. Are there cues such as tone of voice, word phrasing, etc., that remind them of these past events or feelings? Is there an emotional charge when they now experience these cues that perhaps triggers old thoughts and emotional responses?

USING THE TOOLS
Exploring Your Cognitive Map

Are there family myths surrounding your birth and early childhood (e.g., words describing you as a difficult birth, intentional/unintentional pregnancy, wrong gender, cranky temperament, beautiful baby, smart, slow, etc.)?

1. What are the exact words used to describe you as an infant, child, and teen?
   _____

2. What were the circumstances of your caregiving (e.g., breast/bottle fed, daycare, parents worked)?
   _____

3. How many siblings did you have and what was your birth order?
   _____

4. Were you adopted, raised by others than your parents, or did you live in foster care for any length of time?
   _____

5. Did either parent pass away while you were growing up?
   _____

6. What, if any, significant events occurred during the first 5 years, 5 to 10 years, 10 to 18 years of your life (e.g., family moved, went to hospital, went on vacation, death of someone close)?
   _____

7. What are your earliest memories? Are they pleasant or not so pleasant? Which stand out the most?
   _____

8. How would you describe your emotional interactions with each parent and sibling as an infant/toddler, when in primary/secondary school, as a teen, and as an adult?
   _____

9. Were there conflicts with any of the people in the above questions? How were they managed?
   _____

10. What are some of the exact words used in your communications with each in the above two questions?
    _____

Note: These 5 pages may be reproduced by the purchaser for clinical use.

From: Anna B. Baranowsky, J. Eric Gentry, & D. Franklin Schultz, *Trauma Practice: Tools for Stabilization and Recovery.* © 2011 Hogrefe Publishing

11. With whom were you closest? Why?
    _____

12. With whom were you the most distant? Why?
    _____

13. Were you treated with respect and dignity? If not, who did not?
    _____

14. Was anyone psychologically intrusive as you were growing up (e.g., head games, double messages, your feelings used against you, felt like you were not safe in your own mind)?
    _____

15. What is your current relationship with the above persons?
    _____

16. How did your parents discipline you? Under what circumstances?
    _____

17. What were your responsibilities as a child (chores, taking care of siblings, etc.)?
    _____

18. Were you ever left alone for periods of time?
    _____

19. Were you ever frightened? What caused it? How did you and others respond to your fright?
    _____

20. Were you ever in serious trouble at home, school, or elsewhere? What were the circumstances and outcomes?
    _____

21. What were your friends like? Were they allowed to visit you in your home? Why or why not?
    _____

22. How did your parents interact with your friends?
    _____

Note: These 5 pages may be reproduced by the purchaser for clinical use.

From: Anna B. Baranowsky, J. Eric Gentry, & D. Franklin Schultz, *Trauma Practice: Tools for Stabilization and Recovery.* © 2011 Hogrefe Publishing

23. Did your peers ever make fun of you or treat you in a disrespectful manner?

24. How would you characterize the emotional atmosphere of your home (warm, tense, edgy, quiet, calm)?

25. What were holidays like? Birthdays?

26. How were gifts given in your childhood? Were there strings attached?

27. How and from whom did you receive recognition?

28. Were your parents ever divorced? More than once? With whom did you live?

29. Did you have step-parents? What was your relationship with them like?

30. Did either parent have a relationship with or live with a person to whom they were not married? What was your relationship with them like?

31. Did either parent have a previous family? What was your parents' relationship with that family like? What was your relationship with them like?

32. How did your parents communicate with each other?

33. Was there conflict? How did that look (e.g., passive, aggressive, violent, yelling, hitting, threatening)? Under what circumstances? What did you do when conflict occurred?

34. How did your parents demonstrate love to each other, your siblings, you, others? Under what circumstances? Were there favorites? How did that manifest?

Note: These 5 pages may be reproduced by the purchaser for clinical use.

From: Anna B. Baranowsky, J. Eric Gentry, & D. Franklin Schultz, *Trauma Practice: Tools for Stabilization and Recovery.* © 2011 Hogrefe Publishing

35. Was either parent unfaithful? How did you know? What was the result?
   _____

36. Did your parents use alcohol or drugs? Was it a problem? How did it manifest?
   _____

37. Was either parent absent for long periods?
   _____

38. Were your parents outspokenly biased or prejudiced? How did that manifest?
   _____

39. Was either parent psychologically impaired? How so? Physically? How so?
   _____

40. Did you have physical or psychological problems? How were they addressed?
   _____

41. Would you consider either parent abusive (emotionally, physically, sexually)?
   _____

42. Have you experienced any form of abuse (emotional, physical, sexual) from family members or others?
   _____

43. Were you ever touched in a way that left you feeling uncomfortable?
   _____

44. Were you ever stared at or had comments made about your body, your development, or your looks in general?
   _____

45. When and how did you learn about sex?
   _____

46. When and how did you become sexually active?
   _____

47. Were you ever subjected to racist remarks or prejudice?
   _____

Note: These 5 pages may be reproduced by the purchaser for clinical use.

From: Anna B. Baranowsky, J. Eric Gentry, & D. Franklin Schultz, *Trauma Practice: Tools for Stabilization and Recovery.* © 2011 Hogrefe Publishing

48. Were comments ever made about your intelligence or your abilities?

49. What were your experiences in school?

50. Did you have learning difficulties? If so, how did family and/or others respond to your difficulties?

51. What was your socioeconomic status?

52. Were you raised in a rural, small town, suburban, urban, or mixed community?

53. Did you work for money as a child? What were the circumstances?

54. What did you do for fun (activities: scouting, church groups, athletics, other)?

55. What was your weight and body build? Was it a problem?

56. Where you anorexic/bulimic, other?

57. Were you athletic?

58. Did your parents participate in outside activities with you? How was that experience?

59. What was your experience leaving home? Were you relieved, sad, anxious, excited?

60. Are there other areas not asked about in these questions that were a problem for you?

Note: These 5 pages may be reproduced by the purchaser for clinical use.

From: Anna B. Baranowsky, J. Eric Gentry, & D. Franklin Schultz, *Trauma Practice: Tools for Stabilization and Recovery.* © 2011 Hogrefe Publishing

Victim Mythology (CR)

Time required: Six structured sessions.
Materials required: Varies depending on the session progression. See Tinnin (1994).
Indications for use: Use when the primary need is to enhance cognitive coping skills in the Reconnection stage of trauma recovery.
Counterindications: Inability to actively self-soothe.

The concept of Victim Mythology was developed by Louis Tinnin, MD, a psychiatrist and professor at the West Virginia School of Medicine. Dr. Tinnin uses this concept to explain the cognitive and perceptual distortions that so often accompany traumatization, especially developmental trauma. In his TRI Model, now referred to as the Instinctual Trauma Response Model or ITT (http://www.traumatherapy.us/treatmentprocess.htm), Dr. Tinnin utilizes six structured sessions to address and resolve this Victim Mythology in both outpatient and inpatient contexts.

Some of the symptoms associated with Victim Mythology include: diminished self-worth and esteem, desire to cause harm to oneself, seeking and perpetuating trauma-bonded relationships, distorted perception of true danger, foreshortened future, obsessive thinking, compulsive behaviors (addiction), fear of intimacy, and immature spiritual development. The ITT Model utilizes several different techniques to complete both a thorough trauma narrative and successful integration of the traumata to resolve intrusive and arousal symptoms. Dr. Tinnin believes that by resolving traumatic intrusions, the patient is much more able to focus upon and intentionally resolve cognitive and perceptual distortions. The six sessions use a combination of cognitive behavioral techniques to address and resolve these distorted thoughts and behaviors. Old patterns and beliefs of Victim Mythology are gently confronted and replaced with new, more fulfilling thoughts and behaviors.

The term *Victim Mythology* was coined by Louis Tinnin (1994) in the development of his treatment model for trauma (Time-Limited Trauma Therapy). Tinnin found that even after a trauma memory was resolved, many survivors clung to their posttraumatic beliefs that the world is a dangerous place and that the self is flawed. Tinnin believes that by helping the client understand the adaptive nature of the beliefs, by helping the client identify this "mythology" as part of the way that they coped with the overwhelming terror, pain, and grief associated with a traumatic experience, and by helping them to develop beliefs and meanings that are more adaptive to present-day life, the client is able to relinquish these traumagenic distortions.

Any therapy that helps the client identify distortions, script new, more adaptive self-talk, and rehearse these cognitions will work well toward helping the trauma survivor relinquish their victim mythology.

Letter to Self (CR)
(Gentry, personal communication, 2002)

Time required: One or more sessions.
Materials required: Paper and pencil.
Indications for use: Use when the primary need is to enhance cognitive and emotional coping skills in the Reconnection stage of trauma recovery.
Counterindications: Unresolved trauma.

Delivery of Approach

This technique is a way to both center oneself and address victim mythology.

1. Have the client write a letter to the self that experienced the event. In the letter they should first make sense in detail of the earlier self's actions and emotions with the understanding they have achieved through therapy.

2. Move the client toward forgiveness of the self for their actions and emotions both during and subsequent to the event.

3. Help the client welcome that self home into an integrated sense of self. This means they begin to incorporate the experiences of that self as valid information.

4. Finally, have the client make a detailed commitment to self-care, outlining their plans to keep themselves healthy and safe.

3. Behavior

A therapist can guide clients through the recovery process and help them think about and talk about their lives differently. Clients can think and talk about changing, but until their behaviors actually change they will not move into a more healthy and balanced lifestyle. For recovery to be fully integrated into their lives, they must *do* things differently. This is accomplished by them taking the initiative to change their own behaviors. Therapists and clients can prepare for life after therapy by discussing a plan to participate in more healthy and useful behaviors. The following technique is just a small example of the various resources useful to that end.

Self-Help and Self-Development (CR)

Time required: One or more sessions.
Materials required: Varies.
Indications for use: Use when the primary need is to enhance cognitive and emotional coping skills in the Reconnection stage of trauma recovery.
Counterindications: None.

There are literally thousands of books, audio/video tapes, organizations, and websites that are designed to facilitate empowerment through knowledge and connectedness for trauma survivors. One of the most important goals of CBT, or any psychotherapy, is helping the client to find their own resources and answers – to become self-sufficient and symptom free.

We note some website addresses for your use below, including David Baldwin's "Trauma Pages," an excellent resource for all things related to trauma and recovery from traumatic events. Feel free to pass these along to your clients!

http://home.earthlink.net/~hopefull/
http://mentalhelp.net/
http://mentalhelp.net/poc/center_index.php?id=353&cn=353
http://www.1stpm.org/
http://www.beckinstitute.org/
http://www.giftfromwithin.org
http://www.lindaland.com/stressbook/page1.htm
http://www.patiencepress.com/
http://www.psychink.com
http://www.ptsd.va.gov/public/indes.asp
http://www.shpm.com/articles/
http://www.shpm.com/articles/trauma/index.shtml
http://www.sidran.org/
http://www.stressfree.com/index.html
http://www.trauma-pages.com/
http://www.traumaprofessional.org

Visit www.traumaline1.com for an online listing of trauma trained clinicians and ressources.

4. Emotion/Relation

Humans are social animals not only by culture and environment, but also biologically. We are genetically programmed to connect to others. As previously discussed, trauma has the effect of preventing us from successfully connecting to others. The process of trauma recovery is not about forgetting what happened and simply forcing ourselves to behave differently. It is about integrating what happened into a personal story of victory and overcoming the obstacles created by trauma. Reconnecting emotionally is the final victory, accomplished by remembering what happened, learning the lessons of sadness, and relearning to fearlessly love. It is a courageous act of intentionally reentering the world of social connection with an open heart and a clear head. The following techniques help clients remember with intention, mourn their experiences with intention, and reconnect with intention.

Memorials (CR)

Time required: Varies.
Materials required: Varies.
Indications for use: Use when the primary need is to enhance emotional and relational coping skills in the Reconnection stage of trauma recovery.
Counterindications: Inability to actively self-soothe.

The goal of memorials is often to make a bridge from the horrific past to the hopeful future. Memorials provide a ceremonial reconnection between those who have experienced great loss or trauma and their communities through acceptance and acknowledgement – a time to offer mutual support, an honoring for those left behind, and a testimony to those no longer present. This is a chance for closure. Memorials offer a moment for sharing positive restorative memories and a time to reinterpret tragic events. All these things can be integrated into a memorial. It can have a powerful and reconstructive quality.

Delivery of Approach

Memorials can take the form of clients participating in prayer circles, erecting monuments, taking down walls, singing together, burying or burning symbols of a traumatic event, or ritualistically divorcing abusers. There are many forms and few absolute rules. Can you recall meaningful memorials you have attended, developed, processed, or heard about?

There are many approaches to "reconnection" memorials. Please use the time during this section to recall or imagine a memorial that you have used, witnessed, or are aware of that seems meaningful to you. Use the space available in this book to describe memorials that you would like to collect for future use.

USING THE TOOLS
Memorials

Take a moment to reflect upon your journey. What parts of your life need to be memorialized? What losses do you need to commemorate so that you can move on? Take a moment to allow yourself to identify these parts of your life, people, things, and beliefs that need to be identified and write a brief memorial to them all.

Note: This page may be reproduced by the purchaser for clinical use.

From: Anna B. Baranowsky, J. Eric Gentry, & D. Franklin Schultz, *Trauma Practice: Tools for Stabilization and Recovery.* © 2011 Hogrefe Publishing

Connections with Others (RE – CR)

Time required: 20 minutes or more for research and a lifetime for implementation.
Materials required: Varies.
Indications for use: Use when the primary need is to establish meaningful connections with others and enhance cognitive and emotional coping skills in the Reconnection stage of trauma recovery.
Counterindications: None.

It is easy to become overly focused on life's demands and forget to include joyful pursuits, but it is often these joyful pursuits that act as buffers to the pressures of our work and life. Engaging in meaningful activities while connecting with others creates a road back to a healthy life filled with new opportunities and choices. It is common to hear from people that they no longer enjoy the activities they pursued at earlier times in their lives. They no longer sing in a choir, play baseball, read poetry, attend a book club, take acting classes, or run marathons. But why not? What is the meaning of all of this hard work and dedication if we are not also ensuring our own well-being? At this stage of Trauma Practice, recovery is part of the picture, and ensuring that we stay on track means investing in today and connecting to our communities and with people around us in shared and meaningful activities.

USING THE TOOLS
Connections with Others

The rules are as follows:

1. Identify two to three activities of interest within the following four domains: physical, intellectual, creative, and spiritual.
2. Ensure that all selected activities occur within a social context with other people.
3. This is an experiment, so keep it fun.
   Stage I: Simply investigate options or activity areas within each domain.
   Stage II: Select one activity from at least three of the four domains to try.
   Stage III: Try the activity.
   Stage IV: If you like it, continue; if not, choose another to try.
   Stage V: Continue moving through your options until you find three or four that you truly enjoy and wish to continue.

For the third phase of Reconnection in the Tri-Phasic Model, here are four connections:

Connections with others

Identify activities that may interest you within each of the four cluster areas that include a social component. Investigate what activities are available in your vicinity, or create your own group. Select two or three items to get involved in at least once each month. Develop your social life and become involved in your community. Decide if a given activity is a good fit for you only after attending at least three or four times. If not, move on to the next.

1. Physical (e.g., walking club, yoga class, bowling)

   _____

   _____

2. Intellectual (e.g., book club, university/college course, astronomy club)

   _____

   _____

3. Artistic/Creative (e.g., painting class, pottery class, scrapbooking)

   _____

   _____

4. Spiritual/Religious (e.g., join a religious church/temple, learn to meditate, volunteer in a homeless shelter)

   _____

   _____

*The key to happiness is realizing that it's not what happens to you that matters,
it's how you choose to respond.*
k.d. harrell

Note: This page may be reproduced by the purchaser for clinical use.

From: Anna B. Baranowsky, J. Eric Gentry, & D. Franklin Schultz, *Trauma Practice: Tools for Stabilization and Recovery.* © 2011 Hogrefe Publishing

Section 5
Integrative & Clinician Self-Care Models

*Opportunities are usually disguised as hard work,
So most people don't recognize them.*
Ann Landers

- Compassion Fatigue
- Pinnacle Program
- Integrative & Self-Care Models

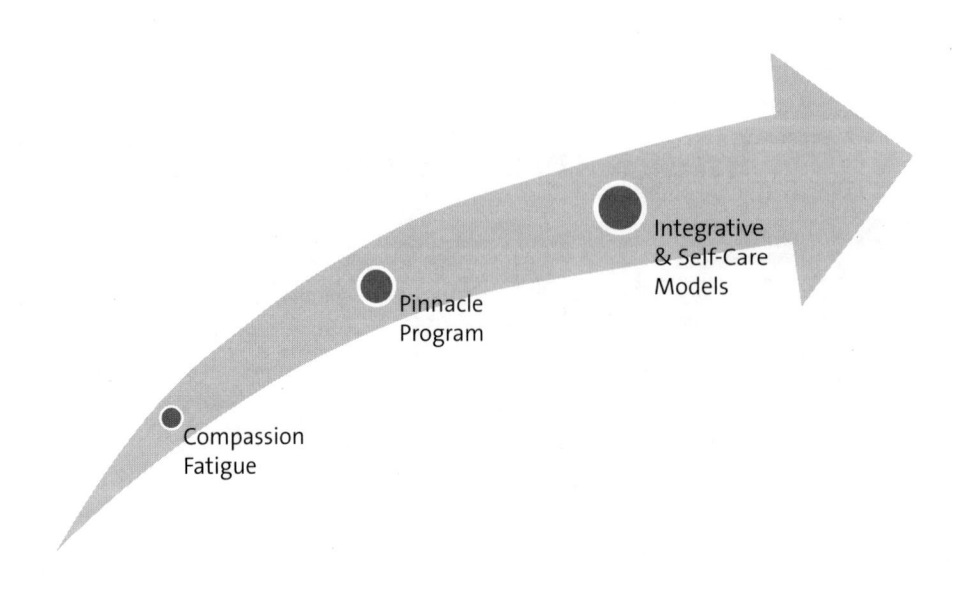

1. The Pinnacle Program: Healing Trauma by Principle-Based Living
2. Compassion Fatigue: The Crucible of Transformation

1. The Pinnacle Program: Healing Trauma by Principle-Based Living

Everyone has his own specific vocation or mission in life; everyone must carry out a concrete assignment that demands fulfillment. Therein he cannot be replaced, nor can his life be repeated, thus, everyone's task is unique as his specific opportunity.
Viktor Frankl

I've been scraping little shavings off my ration of light and I've formed it into a ball and each time I pack a bit more onto it and I make a bowl of my hands and I scoop it from its secret cache under a loose board in the floor and I blow across it and I send it to you against those moments when the darkness blows under your door.
Bruce Cockburn

The Pinnacle Program offers a functional conceptualization of the core Trauma Practice fundamentals because it essentially ties together many of the principles and procedures for trauma recovery within a Tri-Phasic Model. It is possible to utilize this approach both in a proactive self-care strategy as well as an approach to work with client's requiring a semistructured approach and guide to trauma recovery.

Introduction

The Pinnacle Program is a unique combination of accelerated psychotherapy/counseling, performance coaching, and maturational principles designed to help individuals achieve principle-based intentional living while, at once, helping them diminish the symptoms associated with anxiety and traumatic stress. The Pinnacle Program combines the cognitive-behavioral techniques of psychoeducation, self-regulation/relaxation, and *in vivo* exposure (Foa, Keene, & Friedman, 2000; Follette, Ruzek, & Abueg, 1998; Committee on Treatment of Posttraumatic Stress Disorder, National Institute of Medicine, 2008) with intentionality, personal integrity, and internalized locus of control to form an integrated strategy to address the symptoms of anxiety, depression, and traumatic stress. This novel approach allows participants to avoid some of the costs, stigmatization, and disempowerment that are frequently associated with traditional psychiatric treatment.

Instead, it provides a simple path for anyone – but especially survivors of trauma – to engage in a powerful process designed to help turn away from a life dominated by painful symptoms and reactivity toward a healthy and disciplined lifestyle based upon one's own individual purpose and principles. The Pinnacle Program helps participants create, articulate, and rapidly begin living with fidelity to their own "moral compass." By developing this principle-based intentionality, through the principles of self-regulation in the Pinnacle Program, participants enjoy the added benefit of reducing stress-related symptoms. While it may never replace traditional psychotherapy, it does provide a complimentary approach that has effectively accelerated treatment and life satisfaction for scores of clients and hundreds of workshop participants.

The Pinnacle Program was born from a broad, eclectic mix of many ideologies, disciplines, and protocols to form a simple, clear, commonsensical approach to counseling, maturation, and living that helps people migrate from the reactivity of anxiety, depression, and traumatic stress to the comfort and maximal functioning of intentionality. It is rooted in and focused upon helping individuals to live intentionally in the present as a way of rapidly healing their pasts. The methods of the Pinnacle Program are grounded in good CBT (Foa, Davidson, & Francis, 1999; Foa & Meadows, 1997; Friedman, 1996) but without the need of a therapist acting in traditional roles for its application (although participants utilizing the Pinnacle Program in a self-help model *will* need to develop a relationship with another person who they can use as a partner/coach/mentor). Imagine CBT in a homeopathic and humanistic form and you come close to conceptualizing the theoretical underpinnings of the Pinnacle model.

The Pinnacle Program is less a treatment and more a blueprint for living with fidelity to one's individual principles that has the byproduct of symptom reduction. One of the primary components of this model is helping people to understand how their past painful, fearful, and traumatic experiences lead them to perceive a threatening and dangerous world in the present (Holbrook, Hoyt, Stein, & Sieber, 2001). It also helps them to see how present-day intrusions from these difficult past experiences contaminate their current perceptions and cause them to perceive threat where there is none. Helping participants to understand the negative and symptomatic consequences of sympathetic nervous system dominance (see Figure 1) caused by the chronic perception of threat motivates participants to develop an internalized capacity for self-regulation. By intentionally maintaining relaxed bodies in the context of these perceived threats, normally functioning adults can quickly find physiological and psychological comfort, maximize neocortical (thinking) functions, and regain intentional, principle-based behavior, even while confronting these threats (Bremner, 2000; Breslau & Kessler, 2001; Critchley, Melmed, Featherstone, Mathias, & Dolan, 2001; Porges, 1999). In addition, it is well documented that relaxation is a crucial ingredient for the resolution of traumatic stress symptoms and an effective agent in lessening anxiety symptoms (Michenbaum, 1994; Shalev, Donne, & Eth, 1996; Wolpe, 1956).

For all its CBT underpinnings, however, the Pinnacle Program is probably best defined as developmental in its approach to healing trauma because it helps people to restart, continue, and accelerate their natural maturational processes. Painful and traumatic past learning, along with the subsequent adaptations resulting from these traumatic experiences, may cause normal healthy maturation to become thwarted in deference to the constant attention and action that

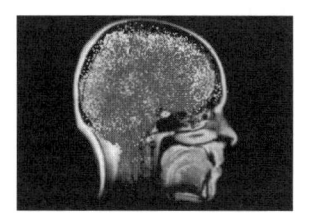

Parasympathetic Dominance	Sympathetic Dominance
• Maximal cognitive & motor functioning	• Compromised cognitive and motor functioning
• Intentional	• Reactive
• Creative problem solving	• Repeating same mistakes
• Transformative leader	• Coercive or hesitant leader
• No trauma or resolved trauma	• Learned through pain, trauma, & fear
• Mobility and decision-making capacity	• Fight/flight
• Muscle relaxation – comfort	• Obsession/compulsion
• Problems = challenge	• Chronic muscle tension
• Peak performance (motor & cognitive)	• Increased threat perception (hypervigilance)
• Intentionally (internal locus of control)	• Diminished brain functioning
• Self-regulatory	• Loss of language & speech (intentional thought)
• Intimacy tolerance	• Intimacy intolerance

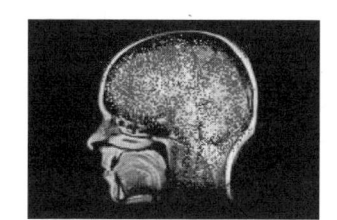

Figure 1. PNS dominance vs. SNS dominance.

perceived threats demand (Bonner & Rich, 1988; Falconer, 2008; Scaer, 2006; Schnurr, Lunney, & Sengupta, 2004). The learning and adaptation that survivors develop from their painful and traumatic history often afflicts them with a heightened perception of threat, even when there is no "real" danger. Depending upon the frequency and intensity of past experiences, these perceptions of threat can frequently be ubiquitous, chronic, and symptom-generating (Spilsbury et al., 2007; Stoppelbein, Greening, & Elkin, 2006).

Once people understand how and begin to regulate the tension in their bodies and calm their nervous systems, they can restart their thwarted natural maturational trajectory (Doublet, 2000; Shusterman & Barnea, 2005). This, in turn, allows them to "get out of the way" of their natural healing processes, leave behind symptoms (Holland et al., 1991), and find satisfying lives based in their own morality, no matter what the external circumstances or conditions (Hamarat et al., 2001). By helping people articulate their intention (i.e., put into words their own mission and morality) and then, simultaneously, helping them relax their bodies when they encounter perceived threats, they are able to begin to live their lives with fidelity to their principles *and* lower their level of stress-related symptoms (Benson, 1997).

The Pinnacle model utilizes three phases, or sections, over multiple weeks:
    Phase I: Education
    Phase II: Intentionality
    Phase III: Practice (Coaching and Desensitization)

These three phases of the Pinnacle Program are developed and thoroughly discussed later in this chapter.

The Pinnacle Program should not be attempted by or with anyone who is experiencing acute psychiatric distress (e.g., suicidal crises, escalating or uncontrollable emotional outbursts, compulsive dangerous or self-destructive behavior, regressive functioning, active addiction, etc.). These individuals should only work with a trained, licensed, and seasoned (i.e., "trauma-informed") professional who can help them become stable enough to utilize this model. Once stabilized, this model can be a wonderful adjunct to ongoing therapy and many therapists will be willing to assist their clients in their movement through the Pinnacle Program's exercises and protocols. The individual who chooses to practice the Pinnacle Program in a self-help format outside of therapy will need to cultivate a relationship with another stable person who can serve as a mentor/coach/accountability partner – much like a "sponsor" in a twelve-step fellowship.

The first phase of the Pinnacle Program is dedicated to psychoeducation – helping the participant to understand traumatic learning, perceived threat, and the ANS. This phase also includes learning the self-regulation skill of relaxing pelvic floor muscles. This important skill helps participants internally attenuate their own level of arousal instead of becoming "stressed out" by the capricious happenings of their lives. By practicing this skill, hundreds of clients and thousands of workshop participants have found that they are able to enjoy comfort in their bodies and remain free from stress no matter the external stimuli.

The second phase of the Pinnacle Program focuses upon helping participants to develop intentionality. This is achieved by first helping them construct their own personal Covenant and a Code of Honor in clear succinct language. The Covenant is the articulation of our purpose for being alive – a personal mission statement. The Code of Honor is a statement of the principles that we choose to govern our lives – each person's individual moral compass. In addition to the construction and sharing of these declarations, the second phase also coaches the individual through exercises designed to assist them in identifying the situations and circumstances where they habitually fail to maintain these principles – instances where they "act out" and breach their integrity. As participants gain the insight to see that reactivity, which leads to the behaviors that breach integrity, is simply the result of allowing the SNS to become and remain dominant after an encounter with a perceived threat, they become increasingly motivated to practice the relaxation strategies of self-regulation when encountering these perceived threats.

The relaxation of self-regulation allows participants to regain comfort, maximal brain functioning, and intentionality in these circumstances and situations, usually within a few seconds (Critchley et al., 2001; Porges, 1999). Said differently, intentional behavior is achieved simply by holding intention in mind while relaxing the body in the context of a perceived threat. The simple elegance of this formula has become the primary engine of change and transformation for the Pinnacle Program.

The final activity of this second phase is facilitating a shift from an external to internal locus of control. After an individual has identified the circumstances and situations where they habitually "act out," this shift is achieved by teaching them to self-regulate by relaxing their bodies (i.e., pelvic floor muscles) so that they can achieve intentionality in these stressful situations while maintaining comfort.

The subsequent work in the Pinnacle Program, which comprises the third and final phase, is essentially the practice of continually confronting "triggers" while maintaining a relaxed body so that participants can become progressively intentional in more and more contexts of their lives. The more practiced at self-regulation an individual becomes, the more they find themselves able to retain fidelity to their Covenant and Code of Honor. Moreover, the more relaxed and intentional (i.e., parasympathetically dominant) a person remains, the fewer symptoms their SNS is generating. In other words, by focusing on intentional living by relaxing while confronting perceived threats, this relaxation will likely lessen many of the symptoms of anxiety, depression, and traumatic stress.

However, almost every client who has successfully completed the Pinnacle Program has found at least one situation (many more for those who have active PTSD symptoms) where, no matter how hard they try to remain self-regulated and relaxed, they still find themselves becoming almost immediately anxious, reactive, and symptomatic. It is hypothesized that this acute reactivity is caused by one or more of their past experiences of traumatic learning intruding into their perceptual system with such intensity that the SNS becomes immediately dominant and brain functioning is rapidly compromised (Herman, 1992; Breslau & Kessler, 2001). These intrusions thwart their ability to self-regulate as the sympathetic nervous system is already strongly compelling them to fight or flight. For those who experience this bewildering inability to self-regulate in particular situations and contexts, they will need to revert to traditional methods of desensitization and reprocessing (exposure, narrative, and relaxation) with a trained professional. They will need to find a therapist who can help them access and desensitize these past painful/traumatic experiences. It should be noted that the primary function and purpose of these traditional methods – Eye Movement Reprocessing and Desensitization (EMDR) (Shapiro, 1995) is most utilized and recommended – is to desensitize and reprocess past experiences sufficiently so that the intrusion of perceived threat is diminished to the level that the participant can now self-regulate in the context of the reminders, or "triggers," associated with these memories. Most clients find, after a few successful sessions of desensitization and reprocessing with past memories, they are better able to keep their bodies relaxed in future situations in which they confront perceived threats associated with these and other memories.

Most clients have found themselves developing a level of proficiency with self-regulation and a modicum of success in confronting and navigating through "stressful" situations with comfort and intentionality within the first couple of weeks of practicing the Pinnacle Program. As they continue to employ self-regulation in the contexts of perceived threats, they often find themselves amazed at the simplicity of maintaining intentionality, comfort, and principle-based living. However, each and every person who has practiced this model will quickly point out that simple is not the same as easy. While it is a simple concept to understand that relaxing one's body in the context of perceived threats yields comfort, maximal neocortical functioning, and

Figure 2. The Pinnacle model

Phase I — Education
- Stress = Perceived Threat
- Autonomous Nervous System
- Fight/Flight = Reactivity = Breach of Integrity

Phase II — Intentionality
- Writing & sharing Convenant and Code of Honor
- Identifying habitual breaches of integrity
- Identifying "triggers"
- Completing Reactive

Phase III — Practice (Coaching & Desensitization)
- Confronting triggers during daily life with relaxation
- Practice increasing awareness and regulation of body ("bodyfullness)

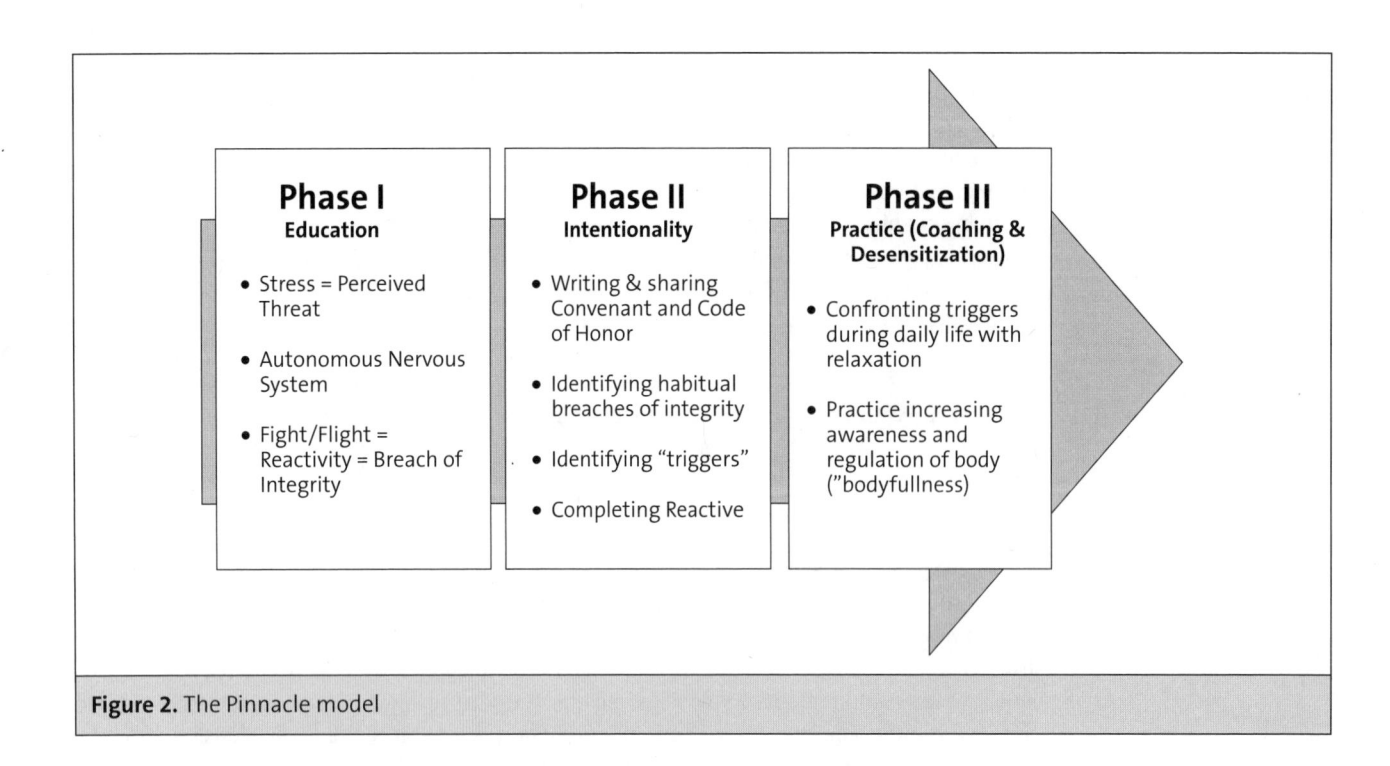

the ability to remain intentional, this capacity also requires constant monitoring and regulation while engaged in the moment-to-moment activities of daily life. Maintaining this state of "bodyfulness" demands ongoing focused attention to areas of the body to which many people have rarely paid attention in the past. Most people find that, as soon as they lose conscious awareness of their pelvic floor muscles, it is not long before those muscles are again clenched and the individual is once again ratcheting upwards toward sympathetic dominance, reactivity, and symptoms.

As previously stated, the Pinnacle model is implemented in three phases or stages (see Figure 2). It is important for individuals engaging in the Pinnacle Program to be stabilized to the degree that they are not experiencing frequent abreactions or suicidal ideation. It is also important to understand that successful outcomes for participating in this program, like all healing, will be primarily contingent upon the quality of the relationship the individual builds with their partner/coach/mentor and the degree to which the individual is able to maintain a positive expectancy (i.e., hope) – that the Pinnacle Program will work for them. To maximize the quality of the relationship and positive expectancy, it is recommended that individuals choose a partner/coach/mentor who has demonstrated the capacity for overcoming difficulty and hardship in their lives. In addition, a partner/coach/mentor should be someone with whom the participant is able to connect and who is able to maintain this supportive connection with warmth, assertiveness, compassion, empathy, and challenge. Ideally, a participant will choose someone who is working this model, or something like it, in their own lives.

Phase I: Education

When working in therapy, this first phase of the Pinnacle Program can usually be completed during a single session. However, the information shared with clients during this first phase will be reviewed and retaught throughout the course of treatment. This is also true for readers practicing the Pinnacle Program in a self-help model outside of traditional therapy formats.

One way that has been effective in transitioning from the well-trodden landscape of traditional psychotherapy into the realm of the Pinnacle model has been to offer participants the following challenge:

Over the next 30 minutes, how would you like to learn how to remain "stress free" when faced with challenges you know you can handle but are leaving you feeling worn, torn, and overwhelmed instead?

(*Note:* This intentionally provocative statement is designed to heighten interest and participation from clients. The clinician is about to embark upon a psychoeducational dialogue with their client to help them to understand that, in the Pinnacle Program, intentional relaxation of the muscles in the body *is* the operational definition of "stress free.")

Most clients cannot resist the temptation to hear how the clinician is going to handle this seemingly impossible task. Even the most recalcitrant clients can usually muster enough willingness and open-mindedness to at least listen, albeit skeptically, for the next half hour. At this juncture clients are asked to identify the sources of stress, or stressors, they perceive in their lives. Most clients recite a litany of objects, people, and activities they believe to be the causes of their stress that might include: finances, relationships, work, traffic, economy, etc. Following the creation of this list of "causes," the therapist can now elicit the "effects" of stress from their client: "What effects are all these stressors having in your life?" The answer to this question is usually a summary list of the symptoms for which the client has sought treatment. Effects such as somatic problems (e.g., headaches, GI disturbances, chronic pain, etc.), anger/irritability, sleep problems, overeating or undereating, substance abuse, relational problems, and anxiety are the more commonly reported effects of these stressors.

Exercise: Take a moment to fill out the table below identifying the causes of stress in your life and then the effects that these stressors have upon you.

Causes and Effects of Stress

Causes	Effects

In therapy, this next step is tricky and needs to be offered with equal parts compassion and humor. The clinician holds up these two lists and, pointing to the lists of "causes," says:

These are NOT the causes of your stress. As long as you believe that these ARE the causes of your stress, there is a good chance you will keep having these (pointing now at the list of "effects").

Occasionally, clients may become a little irritated with this confrontation and the clinician will need to assure them that they have offered this with compassion and ask them for permission to continue to pursue the *real* cause (there is only one) of their stress. Most clients, by this point, are very much engaged and interested in what comes next.

Perceived Threat
↓

Psychological	Brain Mechanics	Other Effects
▲ Heart rate	▲ Basal ganglia & thalmic Fx	▲ Obsession
▲ Breathing rate	▼ Neo-cortical Fx	▲ Compulsion
▼ Breathing volume Centralized Circulation	▼ Frontal lobe activity 　▼ Executive Fx 　▼ Fine motor control 　▼ Emotional regulation	▼ Speed & agility
▲ Muscle tension	▼ Temporal lobe activity 　▼ Language (Werneke's) 　▼ Speech (Broca's)	▼ Strength
▲ Energy	▼ Anterior Cingulate	Constricted thoughts & behaviors
▲ DIS-EASE		Fatigue

↓

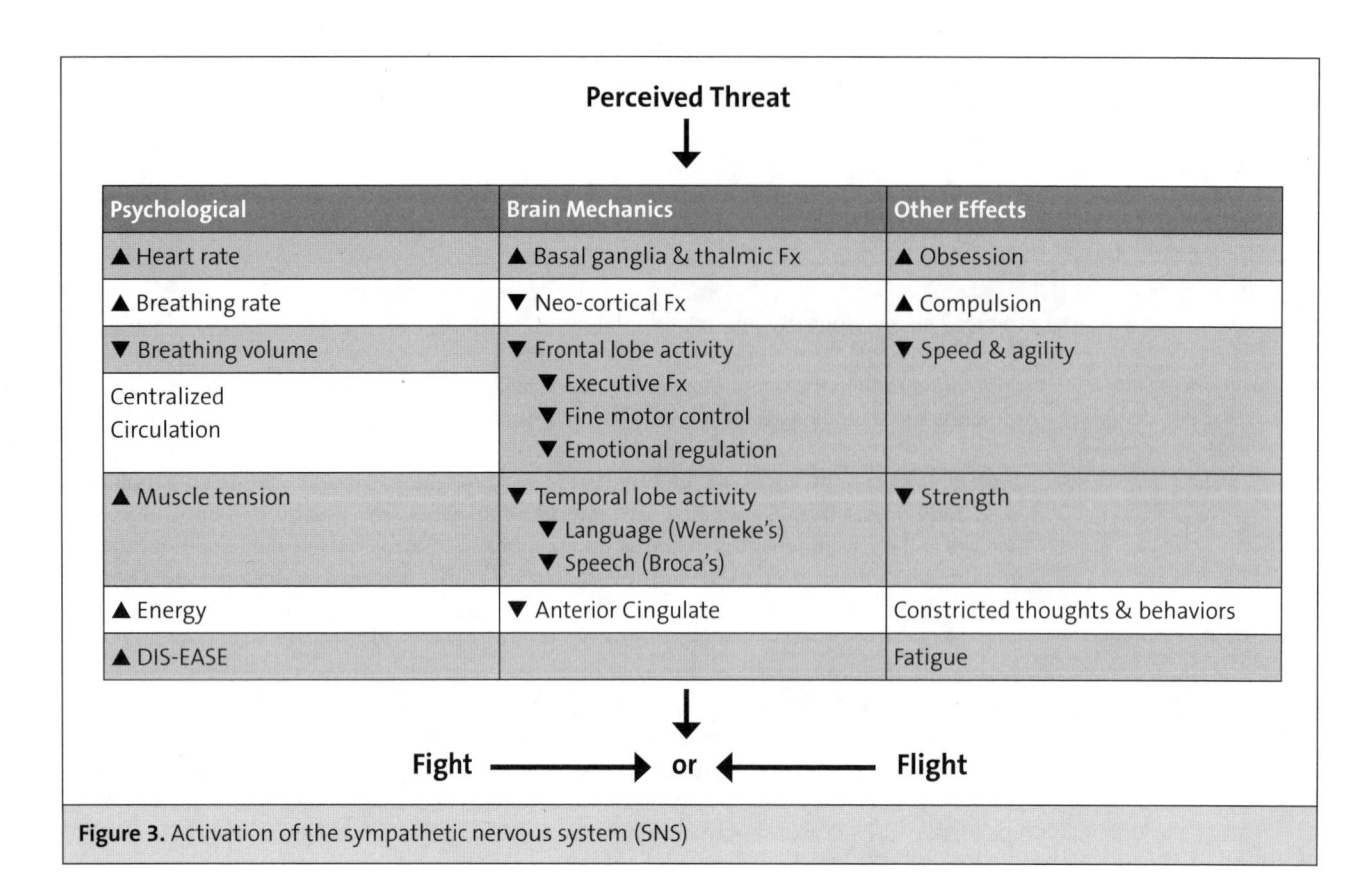

Fight ⟶ or ⟵ **Flight**

Figure 3. Activation of the sympathetic nervous system (SNS)

The next important step is to reveal the true cause of stress which is: *stress = perceived threat*. Perceived threat is the single cause of all stress in human beings. The reason that we experience stress when we encounter financial or relational difficulties or when we are at work or in traffic is because we have learned, through painful or fearful past experiences, to perceive threat in these circumstances. Stress is simply our body and mind's reaction to a danger (Cox, 1992; Hamarat et al., 2001). It makes no difference in our response whether this danger is real or only perceived. Perceived threat (real or imagined) activates the SNS and a discussion about the changes that take place in the body and brain when the SNS becomes activated is the next step of this first phase of the Pinnacle Program (see Figure 3).

When we perceive threat, our SNS activates. These periods of perceived danger are the only time that our SNS will activate and, if we stay in the context of the perceived threat, the SNS will remain activated to become dominant (Yartz & Hawk, 2001). When we do not perceive threat, or when we intentionally relax our bodies, our PNS becomes and remains dominant (Carlson, 2007).

Parasympathetic dominance may best be described as being "comfortable in our own skin" or "fat and happy." The physiological hallmarks of *sympathetic* dominance include increased heart and respiration rate, decreased peripheral circulation, muscle tension, and increased energy (Sapolsky, 1997). In addition to the physiological changes that occur when we perceive threat, our brain also changes (Critchley et al., 2001; Porges, 1999; Scaer, 2006). The middle part of our brains (thalmas), our brain stems, and basal ganglia – often referred to as the "reptilian brain" – activates concomitantly with the SNS when we perceive threat. While in the context of a perceived threat – real or imagined – these parts of our brain become dominant, and while these "reptilian" parts of our brain are becoming dominant, the neocortex, or "thinking" part of our brain, is becoming recessive. The neocortex includes the frontal lobe, the temporal lobe, and the anterior cingulate. These structures have been demonstrated to be the housing for our higher and "executive" functions (Goldberg, 2001). These functions include:

judgment, reason, discernment, fine motor control, identity, time management and conceptualization, language, speech, and the ability to discriminate between real vs. perceived threat. By application, we begin to see that the longer we spend in the context of a perceived threat (real or imagined) without relaxing our bodies, the more we compromise functioning of most of what is human in our brains. We become progressively less able to think clearly and rationally, compromised in our language and memory skills, less agile and graceful, unable to creatively solve problems, and incapable of "being ourselves" when we remain in the context of a perceived threat without relaxing our bodies. Before we give the SNS a bad name and black eye, however, let us examine some of the benefits of sympathetic *activation* (remember activation vs. dominance). The SNS gives us energy and strength, helps us to focus, supplies excitement, and affords us with joy, anticipation, and ecstasy. That is a lot of good stuff. It is only when the SNS gets stuck in the "on" position that it causes problems (Sapolsky, 1997; Scaer, 2006). We can imagine ourselves as automobiles and recognize that we are meant to idle at less than 1000 RPM (PNS), cruise at 2500 RPM (balanced PNS + SNS), and occasionally move up into the higher registers of RPM when we need to pass another car or get somewhere in a hurry (SNS). However, many of us who chronically perceive threat and do not intentionally and regularly relax our bodies are like cars that have the accelerator pedal mashed to floor, in gear, with another foot on the brake. We are spending our days with our RPMs "redlined," going fast but getting nowhere while we burn out the components of our engines. Increasing amounts of research point to this phenomenon as a cause for many diseases and immune dysfunctions (Rothschild, 2000; Scaer, 2006; van der Kolk, 1996)

How did this happen? Good question. The World Health Organization (2007), in a recently published research article, indicated that in high-income countries (North America, Europe, some of Asia, some of South America), we are the "safest" generation to ever live. We are less likely to personally become a victim of warfare, pestilence, famine, disease, disaster, crime, and several other indices of safety than any previous generation. With "Threat Level: Orange" and the never-ending parade of trauma across the evening news, it does not "feel" very safe though, does it? While we may indeed be the safest generation to walk the planet, we also seem to be the most afraid. What is different about our generation than any preceding it? The media. We bear witness to exponentially more trauma and traumatic occurrences than did any of our ancestors through constant bombardment from the media. In 1990, Laurie Pearlman and Linda McCann, in their landmark work with vicarious traumatization, demonstrated that we do not need to be the survivor of a traumatic event to become traumatized – we need only witness it.

To illustrate this phenomenon, I often ask participants in workshops: "How many of you in this room have ever been attacked in a parking garage?" Usually no one raises their hand. If someone does, I ask them to sit out on answering the next question: "How many of you find yourself on-guard and anxious when you are in a parking garage?" It is almost always unanimous that all the hands in the room go up. When asked why they experience this anxiety, you can almost see the light bulb switch on as I hear answers like: "the evening news," "CSI," "the newspaper," "my friend was attacked." These people "witnessed" trauma in a parking garage and the next and future times they found themselves in that context they perceived threat in a parking garage – where there was no real danger. Add to this the phenomenon of state-dependent learning teaching us each and every time that we experience something painful, fearful, or uncomfortable there is a good possibility that we will perceive future situations that remind us of this original event as threatening. Said differently, if we are the *survivor* of a significantly traumatic experience (abuse, rape, natural disaster, motor vehicle accident, etc.), we are more likely to perceive generalized threat in the future. If we are the *witness* to a traumatic event, through the media, hearing stories, reading, or however we learn about something traumatic happening to someone else, we are likely to perceive threat and be afraid in situations that are similar to those we witnessed but happened to someone else. And, finally, if we *experience* painful, fearful, or uncomfortable incidents in our lives, through the process of association, we are likely to perceive threat in situations that remind us of these occurrences (e.g., putting our hands on a hot stove, receiving criticism, encountering periods of financial hardship). All these learning experiences have the potential to cause us to perceive threat in the present where there is no danger. Again, the SNS does not care whether the threat is real or imagined – it will activate in either instance. If we stay in the context of this threat (e.g., parking garage), without intentionally relaxing our bodies, our SNS will become dominant and we will begin to experience the array of symptoms generated by the SNS (e.g., anxiety, panic, difficulty concentrating, irritability, somatic discomfort, etc.). It does not take much insight into this process before we begin to see that, for many of us, threat perception is ubiquitous and chronic, occurring hundreds or thousands of times each day.

The original goal of the SNS was to survive – to help our ancestors recognize and rapidly respond to threat. However, over tens of thousands of years, we humans have developed a frontal lobe that has given us the capacity for reasoning and discernment. Without the capacities of a neocortex, it is imperative that an animal recognize and respond to every threat for its survival since it cannot tell the difference between a real and a perceived threat. However, once we are able to discern this difference, it is no longer imperative, or even useful, to respond to *perceived* threat with an SNS response. There is data to support the compromise of important capacities and skills when the SNS is dominant for extended periods of time. In addition to diminished cognitive and language skills, we can also lose strength, agility, and speed. Any athlete or performance artist will confirm that their best performances occur when they are relaxed and PNS dominant. And any martial artist will also confirm that they are better prepared to protect themselves and disable an attacker when they are also relaxed.

What is RIGHT ACTION, the right use of your will, when you perceive a threat but are in no danger?

Answer: *relax* your body. This is the most important question that you will ever be asked because from the "right" answer to this question flows intentionality, comfort, and maximal performance. In workshops, I often hear participants tell me that right action is to change our perception and I whole-heartedly agree. However, it is nearly impossible to change perception when the SNS is dominant due to diminished neocortical functioning. So, it is best to relax our bodies for 20 – 30 seconds and allow our SNS to dissipate and the frontal lobe to engage so that we can: (a) be comfortable in our bodies; (b) maximize our intelligence and bring to bear all our past learning (i.e., change perception); and (c) shift from reactive fight-or-flight behaviors to intentional and principle-based actions.

Intentionality vs. Reactivity

If we continue to perceive threat without relaxing our bodies, then our SNS will become and remain dominant, flooding our body with energy and chemicals (Yehuda, 2001). All that muscle clenching, heart racing, and shallow breathing is compelling us toward one of the two inexorable goals of the SNS – fighting or fleeing (Cox, 1992; Sapolsky, 1997). With the SNS dominant, we are increasingly compelled to fight or flee *and* we are continuing to gradually lose neocortical functioning (Critchley et al., 2001; McNaughton, 1997; Shusterman & Barnea, 2005). As this energy continues to ratchet upwards with our neocortical functioning continuing to lessen, we will soon find ourselves acting in ways we do not want to act – compulsively and against our will (Takahashi et al., 2005: Yartz & Hawk, 2001). As an example, consider the situation where someone criticizes us at a meeting and we perceive this criticism as a threat (later we will explore and make "good sense" of why we perceive these threats during seemingly innocuous occurrences and while we are perfectly safe). Our face flushes, fists clench, and jaws tighten as we think of several ways to defend ourselves. We decide to say nothing, thinking that it is best to just allow the remark to pass, choosing instead to remain focused on the content of the meeting and compassionate toward our coworkers. However, we notice that we are still uncomfortable (e.g., flushed face, clenched fists, tight jaw) as we become progressively irritated by the remark that occurred a few moments ago. Continuing to perseverate on the comment (therefore remaining in the context of the perceived threat), our SNS continues to ratchet upward while, at the same time, we are losing frontal and temporal lobe functioning. Presently, while still in the meeting, we find ourselves targeting angry looks and making sniping comments towards the offender (fight). After the meeting is over, we find ourselves actively avoiding contact with this person for days, weeks, months, or even years (flight). What happened? Our intention was to simply ignore the critical comment and stay true to our intention of being compassionate, tolerant, and attendant to our work. We did not want to get drawn into these interpersonal politics and we certainly do want to develop and maintain resentment, knowing that it is causing us more harm than anyone else. However, it felt as though we were powerless to stop ourselves even with our best effort.

This concept is the central pillar of the Pinnacle model – helping people to understand and make "good sense" of why they act as they do and then helping them to transform from entrenched, reactive, fight-or-flight behaviors to principle-based intentionality with comfort in their bodies. Those of us who choose to live lives of intention quickly learn that strife and willpower are rarely effective tools toward facilitating this transformation. In the example above, with which most of us can resonate, a *threshold* was crossed and we became compelled, against our will, to fight or flee (see Figure 4). When we have lost too much of our neocortical functioning and we are compelled to act due to SNS dominance, we can no longer hold on to our intention and we instead become compelled to protect ourselves from the perceived threat. We "act out," against our will, with the SNS now in control. We say things we do not mean, we hurt those we care about, we isolate, we overeat, we overspend, we drink and/or use drugs, and we engage in other forms of self-destructive behaviors to either run, fight, and/or soothe the discomfort of SNS dominance. All behavior directed by the SNS will have the goal of either getting away from or neutralizing the perceived threat. Again, it does not matter if the threat is real or perceived. As long as we continue to perceive a threat without relaxing our bodies, we are destined for reactive behaviors. Worse yet, prior to acting out against our principles and breaching our integrity, we will have endured several moments to several hours of uncomfortable SNS dominance. This is the very definition of being stressed out.

Anytime you have acted against your will, breached your integrity, or done anything of which you are ashamed, you probably engaged in these actions while your SNS was dominant

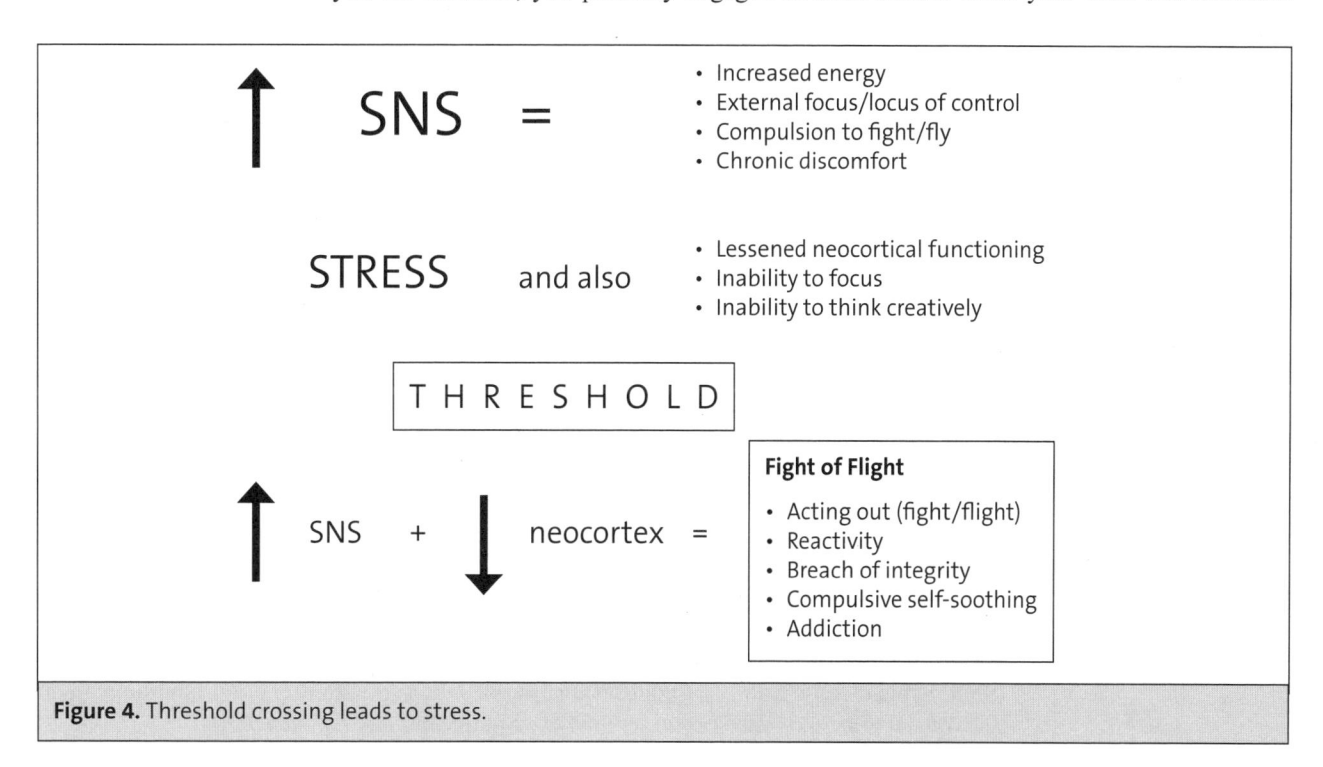

↑ SNS =
- Increased energy
- External focus/locus of control
- Compulsion to fight/fly
- Chronic discomfort

STRESS and also
- Lessened neocortical functioning
- Inability to focus
- Inability to think creatively

THRESHOLD

↑ SNS + ↓ neocortex =

Fight of Flight
- Acting out (fight/flight)
- Reactivity
- Breach of integrity
- Compulsive self-soothing
- Addiction

Figure 4. Threshold crossing leads to stress.

(Takahashi et al., 2005). It is likely that these behaviors were, in some form, an attempt to achieve safety from a perceived threat (rarely a "real" one) by fleeing or fighting. Clients who have participated in the Pinnacle Program found early in their work that they were frequently acting in ways that they did not want to act. They were fighting with spouses they loved, yelling at children they cherished, and dreading work they had chosen as their mission. They learned that many, if not all, of the myriad of symptoms they were experiencing were a result of chronic sympathetic dominance. In my own experience, working with thousands of clients, I have come to embrace the bias that *all* the symptoms my clients report to me are caused by one of two sources: – organicity (something wrong structurally or biochemically) or chronic sympathetic dominance. For those whose symptoms are caused by some organic cause – a structural anomaly or biochemical imbalance – they will usually need some form of organic treatment (e.g., surgery, medication, diet, lifestyle change, etc.). They may still benefit from psychotherapy, but it may be insufficient when the cause of the symptoms is organic in nature.

For those clients whose symptoms are a result of chronic SNS dominance, there is much hope. Human beings (with the possible exception of those with antisocial personality disorder) cannot live in chronic breach of their integrity without suffering symptoms. People who are the most symptomatic also seem to live in frequent betrayal of their mission and their principles. They breach their principles and fail to maintain intentional behavior because they have failed to relax their bodies in the context of perceived threats. As we teach our clients to develop and maintain relaxed bodies in the context of perceived threats, not only do they begin to find themselves able to maintain their principle-based behavior – being the people they intend to be – they also find themselves becoming progressively less symptomatic. They are prohibiting SNS dominance and are instead enjoying the relaxed comfort of PNS dominance, no matter the external situation or circumstance. Intentional, principle-based living achieved through relaxation in the context of perceived threats lessens our nonorganic symptoms.

> **Clinical Note:**
> Clinical professionals who wish to facilitate clients' navigation through the Pinnacle Program will want to develop this previous material into language that is comfortable for themselves and their clients. Having mentored several clinicians through the process of becoming adept with the Pinnacle model, I have discovered that it takes some time to develop mastery with this complex information. It is recommended that readers take some time to familiarize themselves with the literature in the bibliography, speak with experts in the area of human nervous functioning and disorders, and practice for themselves these principles; 6–12 months is a common period required to gain mastery with the psychoeducational concepts and ideas of the Pinnacle model.

Self-Regulation

The final component of the Educational Phase of the Pinnacle Program is teaching self-regulation (Gentry, 2002; Perry, 2007). The use of the term *self-regulation* is different from *relaxation*, even though relaxation is a crucial part of self-regulation. Self-regulation, for use in the Pinnacle Program, is defined as the process of sufficiently and immediately relaxing and keeping relaxed one's body so that the SNS does not achieve dominance. This means an individual must develop sufficient mastery of a set of relaxation skills that they can implement at any time to shift from SNS to PNS dominance – regardless of the external circumstance or situation. In addition, it also requires that they develop the capacity to monitor themselves for SNS activation and then implement these relaxation strategies to prevent the SNS from achieving dominance. Said differently, self-regulation is the development and ultimate mastery of the ability to internally attenuate our own level of arousal, anxiety, and stress (i.e., SNS dominance) to a level of comfort that facilitates maximal neocortical functioning and intentional principle-based behavior. Said even more simply: *Stop clenching*.

Traditional relaxation approaches employed in the service of mental health treatment have proven useful, but require attention and dedication and are not always immediately effective with every individual. Maintaining a relaxed and comfortable body while engaged in the activities of daily life, especially when those activities involve frequently confronting perceived threats, is extremely challenging. Progressive relaxation, paradoxical relaxation, meditation, autogenesis, and even diaphragmatic breathing all require the client to disengage from their current activities to some degree while they attempt to bring about relaxation by one of these methods. This disengagement makes concurrent sustained attention on work or other activities of daily living extremely difficult. These methods work wonderfully when a person has ample time and space to engage in these deeper relaxation protocols (Jamison, 1996). It is recommended to individuals who practice these and other methods to continue their practice. However, the Pinnacle Program asks them to add the skill of self-regulation to their toolkits.

Self-regulation, as defined and employed in the Pinnacle Program, is simple, but not easy. It involves a commitment to life-long practice of developing and maintaining relaxation of the pelvic floor muscles (i.e., psoas, sphincter, and pubio-coccyx or "Kegel" muscles). The muscles of the pelvic floor and, more specifically, the psoas muscles have been gaining attention as an important area for the regulation of anxiety and stress (Bercelli, 2007, 2009; Heim et al., 1998; Krost, 2007). I have called this ongoing identification and regulation of muscle tension *bodyfulness*. Whereas "mindfulness" challenges the client to disengage from trying to control thoughts and just notice them while attempting to relax, the "bodyfulness" of self-regulation asks the client to not attend to thoughts at all, but instead maintain an awareness and relaxation of their pelvic floor muscles (Jamison, 1996; Kabat-Zin, 1990). Relaxation of the pelvic muscles can bring about an immediate and profound relaxation of the entire body – often within 20–30 seconds. Slower and deeper breathing, reduced heart rate, relaxed core and peripheral muscles, and reactivation of neocortical function are all benefits of a relaxed pelvic floor (see Figure 5). It is difficult, if not impossible, to generate the visceral effects of fear and SNS (e.g., elevated heart rate, clinched muscles, shallow breath, diminished cognitive functioning) when the pelvic muscles remain relaxed. In other words, if you can keep the muscles between your waist and thighs relaxed and unclenched, the rest of you will likely be comfortable and PNS dominant, no matter what is happening around you. I have had reports from many clients, before they learned pelvic floor relaxation, who were so phobic or scared that they could not engage in certain activities (flying, driving over bridges, getting shots, and even skydiving). As they learned and began practicing self-regulation, they were able to engage in these activities and reported that they had no sense of discomfort or fear. Probably

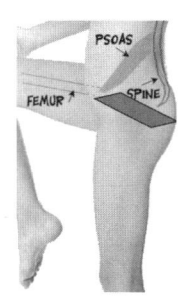

- Relaxing tension of pelvic floor muscles switches from sympathetic to parasympathetic dominance
- Psoas, Spincter, and "Kegels" (anterior + posterior)
- Regaining of neocortical functioning in 20–30 seconds
- Relieves pressure on vagus nerve
- Difficult, if not impossible, to experience stress – comfortable in one's own skin

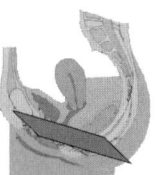

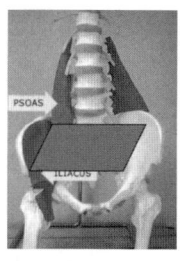

Figure 5. Self-regulation by relaxation of the pelvic floor muscles.

the most important point about pelvic floor relaxation as a strategy for self-regulation is that people can do it while they are engaged in other activities. It takes practice and determination, but after a few months, most clients who have practiced this method find that they can effectively attend to the dialectic of relaxing their pelvis while engaging in work, performance, school, relational encounters, and the other activities of life. However, pelvic floor relaxation never seems to become automatic and requires constant attention, or bodyfulness. Individuals wanting to remain comfortable, maximally functioning, and intentional will need to willfully practice this simple skill of pelvic relaxation moment-to-moment for the rest of their lives. It is simple, but not easy.

Why does the relaxation of the pelvic floor muscles result in profound systemic relaxation that affects both body and brain? We are not certain. I discovered this technique from emergency medical technicians (EMTs) when I learned their protocol for assisting a person who is suffering an attack of tachycardia, or dangerously fast heart rate. Paramedics are taught to use a process that is called a *val salva* manoeuver that triggers a *vaso-vagal* response (Lim et al., 1998; Waxman et al., 1980). This response is accomplished by having the patient "bear down," with a gentle downward and outward pressure, as though they are having a bowel movement. This action, in most patients, produces a significantly precipitous bradycardic (slowed heart rate) response within a few seconds (Kinsella & Tuckey, 2001). This response is known to occasionally cause heart attacks with geriatric patients when they go to the bathroom (Sikirov, 1990). I became increasingly curious how manipulation of the configuration of the muscles in one's pelvis could have such a profound effect upon heart rate. Although I have been able to find little information or data regarding these muscles and the effects they have, except in the area of incontinence, the information I have found has led to the vagus nerve (Porges, 1992). The vagus nerve is the tenth cranial nerve. It is the longest nerve in the human body; hence its name – *vagus* is Latin for "wanderer." It is connected to the roof of our mouth, follows the carotid artery into the chest and terminates at the perineum (where the legs join together). The vagus nerve is intricately connected to the regulation of the PNS and the SNS; it controls and/or regulates many of these functions in both our bodies and our CNS. We know vagal nerve stimulation can and does have a profound effect on mood and is a growing treatment for some of the most recalcitrant mood disorders. We also know that mild manipulation of the vagus nerve can cause a person to pass out or have extreme heart rate variability. It has also has been linked to paralysis (i.e., conversion disorder) and dissociation (George et al., 2000) during periods of extreme stress.

We have much to learn about the vagus nerve and, after multiple attempts of scouring the literature, I have been unable to find any articles that give a satisfactory explanation for the mechanics and relationship between pelvic floor relaxation, the vagus nerve, and PNS vs. SNS dominance. I am unable to provide a good citation that supports the notion that when you relax your pelvic muscles then the rest of your body relaxes and you are able to think clearly and act intentionally. I do, however, invite you to try it. If it works for you, then you may wish to continue to utilize it as a method for self-regulation. It will certainly cause no harm. Scores of clients and thousands of workshop participants have reported to me that the quality of their lives transformed from practicing this simple skill of relaxing their pelvic muscles when they experience perceived threat. Comfort, maximal functioning, and intentionality follow in its wake.

A detailed explanation of self-regulation, SNS vs. PNS dominance, and the procedure for pelvic floor relaxation is contained in Appendix 1: Self-Regulation. I make copies of this handout available to all my clients and workshop participants. Please feel free to copy and disseminate this handout. It is recommended that you practice the exercise contained in the handout and complete 30 seconds of totally relaxing your pelvic floor muscles. When you have completed the 30 seconds, notice how you feel. You will likely notice that you are comfortable, sleepy, relaxed, your breathing will have slowed, and the muscles elsewhere in your body will have released. For those people having some difficulty establishing a "felt sense" of their pelvic floor muscles (anecdotally, this is about 10% of the clients and workshop participants), I do a "Kegel exercise" with them (Kegel, 1951). This is done simply by asking a person to tighten, for 5 seconds, the muscles they would use if they wanted to stop urination midflow. Tighten these muscles as tight as you can for the 5 seconds and then release with a deep breath. Take a second deep breath and then release these muscles even more profoundly. I ask participants to then memorize this sensation of pelvic relaxation and to replicate it anytime they feel tense, perceive a threat, or are aware of any stress in their bodies. For those that continue to have difficulty establishing a "felt sense" of their pelvic muscles, I will refer them to a message therapist, a neuromuscular therapist, or an osteopath and tell them to ask for help in locating their psoas and "Kegel" muscles. A good practitioner of kinesiology will be able to help you locate and release these muscles.

Clinical Note:
When working with clients at the conclusion of this session of treatment, and after a client has been able to successfully get and keep their pelvic muscles relaxed for a short period of time, I congratulate them on learning one of the most important skills they will ever learn. Before they leave the session I playfully ask them the following question:

So, are you leaving this session knowing how to never experience stress again ... for the rest of your life.

From most of my clients I get a grumble, a smile, and something like: "Yeah, but I didn't know it was going to take this much work." As they leave the session, I take heart knowing that I have given maximal attention to both the therapeutic relationship and positive expectancy – the two most powerful predictors of positive change. They (and now you also) have been equipped with powerful and necessary information to help them live lives of comfort and intention.

Whether it takes one or two sessions to complete this Educational Phase of the Pinnacle Program, with its completion you will likely witness a growing sense of hope and anticipation from your client. As you reinforce for them the understanding that as they practice relaxing their bodies, in the form of pelvic floor relaxation, they will be able to enjoy immediate comfort, maximal functioning, and be able to live with fidelity to their own principles and morality, it is likely that they will be excited about continuing the work toward developing and maintaining this capacity. With the completion of this phase, I ask my clients to complete, as homework, the Pinnacle Exercises that will help them articulate their Vision, their Covenant, and their Code of Honor. I ask them to find 60–90 minutes of contemplative time where they can work on these exercises without interruption or encroaching demands. A copy of the template for these exercises may be found in Appendix 2. Use the template to construct and complete a statement of your Vision, Covenant, and Code of Honor. You should be as succinct and clear as possible in the completion of this exercise.

For those reading this chapter and wishing to engage in the Pinnacle Program in a self-help model, please read and complete the Pinnacle Exercises contained in Appendix 2. After completing these exercises, you will want to recruit a person and/or a network of people that you can use for support, sharing, and accountability. You will use this person or these people throughout your work with the Pinnacle Program. In selecting your support person/network, it is best to work with others who are engaged in some form of self-healing and actualization – someone who is empathetic and committed to helping you become the person you wish to be. You may decide to begin the Pinnacle Program with a group of others who wish to practice this model of self-help in their lives. The Pinnacle Program lends itself quite well to work in a group format. (*Note:* If you do choose to work within a group, please contact Dr. Eric Gentry via http://www.compassionunlimited.com and assistance in structuring the group will be provided.)

Phase II: Intentionality

Do I go where I aim myself?

- Requires self-regulation
- Mission-driven
- Internal locus of control
- Principle-based
- Tolerance of pain for growth
- Maturation of spirituality

> ***2168 miles. 5,000,000 steps. 2,000 bug bites, 21 blisters, hypothermia, and a stress fracture.***
> In the summer and fall of 1996, I thru-hiked the Appalachian Trail from Mt. Katahdin, Maine to Springer Mountain, Georgia. I spent the first night of the six-month hike at Daisy Pond Shelter, 2.3 miles south on the trail from Mt. Katahdin. It was the first of hundreds of three-sided sleeping shelters that dot the trail about every six miles all the way from Maine to Georgia. I was cold, scared, and alone. I discovered in that shelter, like the hundreds that were to follow, a notebook was maintained for each hiker to write whatever thoughts or information that they would like to leave for future hikers that would pass through the shelter in the days and weeks to come. These notebooks increasingly became an important source of news, entertainment, information, connection, and comfort for every hiker on the trail. Sometimes funny, sometimes sad, and sometimes poetic, these notebooks were savored at the end of the day at each shelter and most days I added my thoughts and feelings to this patchwork narrative. On that first night in that first shelter I opened and read the first page of that first notebook. Here is what it said: *The first step of a journey is great not for the distance it covers but for the direction it heralds.* I lay there that night meditating on this truism – on what a first step declares and the potency of that declaration. After all was said and done, that first step provided me with enough momentum and energy to take the next five million and complete what only 5% of those who take that first step complete – a thru-hike of the Appalachian Trail.

This second phase of the Pinnacle Program focuses first on helping the individual to articulate and share their Vision, Covenant, and Code of Honor. Once you have completed the Pinnacle Exercises and constructed these three documents, it is important that you develop a relationship with one or more individuals who can serve as your coach/accountability partner. You should make a photocopy of your Vision, Covenant, and Code of Honor for your partner. You will be returning over and over again to these documents in future meetings. Now, schedule your first meeting with your partner/mentor/coach.

This first meeting is an important moment in the trajectory of your healing and self-actualization. With the completion of the Pinnacle Exercises, you are emerging – stepping forward as best you can with a declaration of who you are and how you *choose* to be. We will want to lend to this moment all the gravitas that it deserves and you will want to select as a partner to witness this declaration someone who can also extend this reverence. In addition, a few moments spent discussing with your partner the process of writing your Vision, Covenant, and Code of Honor is time well spent. A conversation that includes difficulties, challenges, and triumphs are all worthy of discussion in this early part of the first meeting with your partner.

Next, you can discuss with your partner your experiences with self-regulation. Did you attempt to self-regulate during times of anxiety, stress, and perceived threats? What were the outcomes of these attempts? Do you need some remediation for self-regulation skills?

Section 5: Integrative & Clinician Self-Care Models 141

> **Clinical Note:**
> The comments I most often hear in these early sessions is that my client was able to find comfort, relaxation, and had some minor success *when they remembered to relax their bodies*. However, most will have only practiced self-regulation a few times between sessions. It is important for the clinician to begin with encouragement and good motivational interviewing techniques. One example of this might look like the following: *So, you were able to self-regulate during a few experiences over the past week and you were able to be comfortable in your skin and act like you wanted to?* [Client acknowledges] *Hmm. And when you forgot to self-regulate, you were uncomfortable and "acted out," right?* [Client acknowledges] *Where am I going with this?* This playful confrontation reinforces for the client that they are able to choose to act differently but must do so by remembering to first relax their body instead of trying to "think their way through."
>
> For clients who fail to complete the Pinnacle Exercises, some time should be spent discussing the meaning of this shortcoming. Are they committed? Do they wish to negotiate to complete these exercises for the next or future session? Is there something else more emergent that needs attention? Is there something that is thwarting their belief that they can change? All these are appropriate discussion for those who fail to complete the exercises. For those who articulate a desire to continue but, for whatever reason, were unable to complete the exercises, I help them to complete an abbreviated version of their Covenant and Code of Honor. I ask them to identify three words that best describe their purpose for being alive and then I ask them to identify three words that represent the principles they choose as their own personal code – their moral compass. I then use these six words to help them move through the following exercises of the session.

Appendix 3 contains a worksheet that will assist you in navigating through the concepts, activities and exercises of this second phase of the Pinnacle Program. Contained in the Reactive to Intentional Worksheet are the five main components of this phase of the program. These are:
1. Covenant/Code of Honor;
2. Reactive behavior/breach of integrity;
3. Intentional behavior;
4. Triggers; and
5. Narratives.

This portion of the work in the Pinnacle Program will address each of these five components in relation to one or more reactive behaviors and help you prepare to transform this habitual reactivity into intentional, principle-based behaviors. Please print and have ready to utilize Appendix 3: Reactive to Intentional worksheet for this portion of the work. Figure 6 below is a reproduction of and corresponds with the worksheet.

1. *Covenant/Code of Honor*. Using the worksheet, identify a few principles from your Covenant or Code of Honor that you habitually breach during the course of a day or week. What are the primary points of your moral compass? How do you *want* to act at home, at work, or at school? Write in a few words that define the principle behind your intention (e.g., kind, friendly, helpful). In the example in Figure 6, you can see the example is "Compassionate." We are using for this example the scenario that was discussed earlier in this chapter, during which the subject was criticized in a meeting and then engaged in reactive behavior.

2. *Breach of Integrity/Reactivity*. In this second box, you are asked to identify your reactive behaviors – the instances where you habitually breach either your Covenant or your Code of Honor. This is simply facilitated by selecting one of the tenets of your Covenant or one of the principles of your Code and asking yourself: *Where do I find myself failing to be _____ (compassionate, frugal, honest, trustworthy, kind, etc.)*. I usually offer an example of such a breach from my own life (my Covenant sits framed on a table in my office).

One I frequently share with clients is: *Every morning I wake up and make a petition to be an instrument of love and peace on this planet...then I get behind the wheel of my car* <smile>. *It is hard to reconcile the intention of being an instrument of peace while yelling at someone to get out of my way.* In addition to getting a smile from my client, this disclosure usually helps them understand the look and feel of these instances of reactivity. Another metaphor that is helpful is that of a train on its tracks. The Covenant and Code of Honor are the "tracks" that you have laid that say "this is my path ... this is who and how I choose to be." You are the train, chugging along the rails of your intention. Describing the ways in which you end up "in the ditch" is a helpful aid in understanding reactivity. Whatever way you use is fine as long as you are able to describe the specific behaviors in which you engage that are repetitive, reactive, and represent a breach of your integrity. "Contempt" is identified as the reactive behavior in Figure 6.

3. *Intentional Behavior*. To complete this third box you will need to find behaviors alternative or opposite to your breaches of integrity – behaviors that you would like to practice in the similar situations. These behaviors should be actions that represent fealty to your Covenant and Code of Honor. In the example above, "speaking assertively" to the criticizer represents intentional behavior. This is contrasted with the harboring of contempt that is identified as the reactive behavior that, by engaging, the subject breaches their integrity.

4. *Triggers*. Explaining and helping participants understand and identify their "triggers" may be the most challenging part of the Pinnacle Program. Triggers are the real-world objects or occurrences that we experiences as perceived threats. Triggers can be anything perceived by the five senses – something felt, heard, seen, smelled, or tasted – that activates the SNS. We usually encounter triggers a few seconds to a few minutes before engaging in reactive behavior, although this latency period can be longer. Triggers most often addressed in the Pinnacle Program tend to be relational encounters but they can be anything from an old song to a particular date (e.g., anniversary) or time of day (e.g., bedtime). Triggers are present remembrances, or "little flashbacks," associated with previous experiences of pain, fear, and/or trauma that cause us to perceive threat when we encounter these objects or occurrences. Failure to relax our body in the context of one or more of these triggers leads to SNS dominance that, in turn, leads to reactive behavior and breaches of integrity. We want to begin to recognize our triggers and confront them with pelvic floor relaxation. If we can keep our bodies relaxed during and immediately after an encounter with a trigger, then we can confront

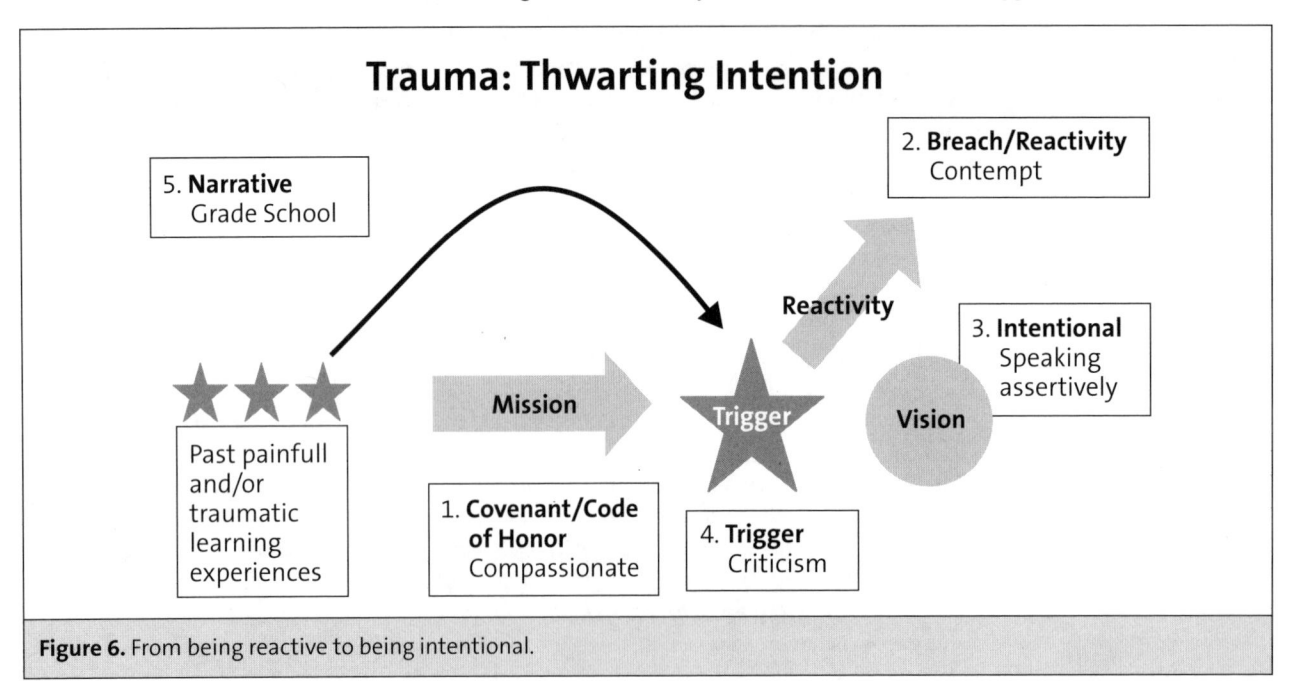

Figure 6. From being reactive to being intentional.

these situations with: (a) a comfortable body without stress; (b) maximal neocortical functioning with creative intelligence for problem-solving; and (c) the ability to maintain intentional behavior where previously we have been reactive.

The best way to discover and confront triggers is by developing an ongoing awareness of (pelvic floor) muscles tension – or "bodyfulness." If our muscles are clenched, then we have encountered a perceived threat. Tracing backwards in time from the moment of awareness of our tightened muscles to find whatever we have encountered that might have been perceived as a threat will help us to grow this capacity for finding triggers. Being reminded that "stress" is caused only by perceived threat and that every time we experience stress during our day we are perceiving some kind of threat (real or imagined) will help us orient toward looking for the triggers that precede and precipitate this perceived threat (see Figure 6). As we develop this capacity for bodyfulness, we begin the transformative process of migrating from an external locus of control in which we are victims of the capricious whims of our environment and circumstances to intentional and principle-based living with internal control of our anxiety and fear.

After encountering a trigger, we find that we have a "window of opportunity" in which we must relax our bodies if we want to maintain intentionality. Depending upon the individual, a few seconds to a few minutes of experiencing sustained threat perception will lead to progressive SNS dominance and diminished frontal lobe functioning. In this state of constriction, we become increasingly compelled to fight or flee while, concurrently, we will experience loss of intention, memory, language skills, and creativity. It does not take long in this condition for us to lose the ability to intervene for ourselves in a productive manner and, once again, we may find ourselves acting out, "in the ditch," and repeating the same mistakes of our pasts. For most people, and I include myself here, it takes a significant number of times of ending up "in the ditch" and harvesting the pain, frustration, and shame that comes from these reactive behaviors before we become willing to apply the simple solution of relaxation to the problem. Said differently, many of us have to fight and struggle with these situations long and hard enough until we have suffered enough pain that we can finally surrender to this simple solution (see Figure 7).

> **Clinical Note:**
> This insight can become a useful motivational tool for later sessions with our clients when we can ask them: *Have you had enough pain yet or do you need some more?* This question should always be attenuated with compassion and loving kindness, not with sarcasm or aggression. However, the judicious use of this question will help underscore for your client that they now have a choice. Whereas they were previously condemned to repeat these same mistakes, they can now choose to relax their body for 20–30 seconds to regain comfort and intentionality.

$$\frac{\text{Perceived Threat} + \text{No Danger}}{} = \text{RELAX}$$

= Comfort in Body
= Increased Thinking Capacity
= Ability to Live with Integrity

Figure 7. Formula for Hope #1

5. *Narratives*. This may be the most exciting part of the Pinnacle Program – helping individuals attach narratives and meaning to their triggers and helping them make "good sense" of their perceived threats. There are good reasons why we perceive threat where there is no *current* danger. The reason that we perceive threat in the present while encountering objects or situations that hold no real danger for us is not because we are crazy. It is because of the intrusion of past painful or traumatic experiences into our present perceptual systems. Any painful past experience, no matter how brief or seemingly innocuous, can erupt into present consciousness and cause us to perceive threat where there is none. There are literally millions of these past experiences by the time we reach adulthood. Add to this fertile and fomenting compost the experiences of secondary traumatic stress we experience through the media, or our work for those of us who are caregivers, and it is obvious that there is an infinite number of potential past experiences that shape the perceptions of objects and activities of our daily adult lives toward that of perceived threat.

Before beginning this process of maturation, most of us, when we encountered a trigger, did one of two things: We tried to either neutralize or avoid the threat. We rarely, if ever, confronted the trigger with relaxed bodies. The cost of this avoidance strategy was that we remained anxious, reactive, and diminished in our functioning every time we encountered these triggers. We became victims of our environment, having to fight or flee to manage stressful circumstances. The hidden costs of this strategy were even greater. Every time we encountered a perceived threat, we experienced a certain level of SNS activation and, if we remained in the context of this threat for a period of time, SNS dominance. Then we employed some form of attack or avoidance. This meant that the level of arousal we experienced when and if we did ever confront a trigger remained high, not ever diminishing because we had not yet successfully relaxed our body in the context of these triggers. A single instance of confronting a trigger with a relaxed body begins the process of desensitization. After the first time of keeping our bodies relaxed throughout an encounter with a trigger (20–30 seconds), the trigger will never again produce as much arousal as it did in previous encounters. The more times we relax in the context of the trigger, by the process of reciprocal inhibition or desensitization, the less intense the arousal will be in subsequent encounters. We become less reactive in our behaviors and more comfortable in our bodies as past experiences have less and less effect upon our present functioning. Said differently, we heal our past by relaxing our bodies in the present. This is a primary transformational engine of the Pinnacle Program: Knowing that we can unchain ourselves from the trauma and painful learning of the past with simple self-regulation.

In the past, when we encountered triggers with SNS dominance and diminished neocortical functioning we were unable to use language very successfully in these situations. We forgot the things we learned, we stumbled over our words, and we experienced a never-ending loop of obsessive, less-than-helpful thoughts. This diminished neocortical functioning, accompanied with the compulsion of the SNS to get us out of danger, preempted any attempts we might have made to understand why we were so afraid when there was no real danger. As we begin to bring relaxation to the equation and remain PNS dominant through an encounter with a trigger, we can begin to ask ourselves: *Why am I so frightened? What experience(s) from my past has/have caused me to perceive a threat in this situation?* We begin to mine the experiences that have led us to perceive threat in the present. We begin to make "good sense" of why we are so afraid. As we are able to make sense and understand why our SNS has become activated and why we perceive threat in the present – honoring the experiences of the past where we learned through pain, fear, and trauma – we begin to experience some compassion and respect for ourselves. We discover that we were not sick or defective; we were simply adapted to a world where pain, fear, and trauma were normative. We are no longer in need of this adaptation and we can begin to let it go, finding comfort, maximal functioning, and intentionality instead.

It has long been understood that imaginal exposure to traumatic memories, paired with relaxation, is an effective treatment for traumatic stress. Almost all effective treatments for posttraumatic stress utilize this construct of reciprocal inhibition – pairing of exposure and relaxation – in some form to facilitate desensitization that helps clients lessen symptoms of posttraumatic stress. Beginning in the late 1980s, we began to see that the type of exposure was important. The construction and sharing of complete chronological narratives of traumatic experiences, paired with relaxation, was more effective than simply talking at random about parts or fragments of the trauma. Helping survivors of trauma construct and share their narratives has a powerful ameliorative effect upon the symptoms of traumatic stress, especially the reexperiencing symptoms (e.g., flashbacks, nightmares, psychological or physiological arousal with cues). The Pinnacle Program creates a simple and naturalistic method for individuals to begin to construct and understand these narratives for themselves. As we practice relaxing our bodies and confronting triggers instead of avoiding them while engaged in the activities of our lives, we can begin to pay attention to the narratives that will begin to spontaneously emerge.

An excellent example of this process is illustrated by an experience with a recent client. A 30-year-old married female, who is employed full-time and also a full-time student, had been in therapy with me for six sessions. Her complaints, upon intake, were uncontrollable crying, compulsive behaviors, and dysthymia, or chronic low-grade depression. We had been navigating through the Pinnacle Program and she reported having some success with pelvic floor relaxation, finding some degree of comfort and ability to be intentional in situations in which she had previously engaged in compulsive behavior. She also reported that she was having difficulty remembering to relax her body, but when she did remember, her quality of life was getting much better. On the seventh session she presented for therapy and reported that her husband was experiencing depression and had spent several days of the past week "on the couch," refusing to look for work or engage in any activities. My client reported that, in the past, this behavior would make her angry and she would attempt to coerce her husband into gainful action. However, this time she said that she sat down with her husband on the couch and said "When I was a child and my mother was depressed and despondent, it meant that I was soon going to be cold, hungry or dirty. I am an adult now. I know that I will not be cold, hungry, or dirty when you are not present with me. I love and desire you no matter what." There were tears in both our eyes as she related this story to me. This experience is a perfect example of the elegance with which clients can find resolution of their painful past without having to engage in regressive therapy to desensitize the memory. Instead, she was able to bring a modicum of healing to her past, present, and future by relaxing her body in the present and practicing intentionality – it was part of her covenant to love and desire her partner no matter what.

Warning:
While the Pinnacle Program offers a self-help process for developing and understanding how our traumatic history has affected our present functioning, participants should remain mindful that uncovering traumatic material always has the potential to be overwhelming and, in some cases, debilitating. It is important for participants of the Pinnacle Program, whether they are currently working with a therapist or practicing this model in a self-help capacity, to create for themselves ample opportunity to regularly share these narratives with their therapist or their coach/mentor/partner. We should share these narratives only with people who have demonstrated *their* capacity to self-regulate and bear witness to the stories of our past without needing to "contaminate" them with their own anxiety. Developing the understanding and the subsequent narratives of our past experiences that have led to perceived threat in the present is only half of the work. The full relief from our traumatic and painful past comes only when we share these experiences with a compassionate and empathic listener. If we are chosen by another to be a listener to their narratives, we will want to listen empathetically but dispassionately. We will not want to be reactive to their stories and instead help them to make "good sense" of why these experiences have caused them to perceive threat in the present while encouraging them to (a) remain relaxed while

> delivering their narratives and (b) self-regulate when they encounter triggers related to these narratives in the future. Finally, if you or someone with whom you are working in the Pinnacle Program becomes acutely symptomatic (i.e., sleep problems, depression, suicidal thoughts, self-destructive behaviors, etc.), do not hesitate to contact a licensed professional familiar with traumatic stress and its treatment for consultation.

This second, or intentionality phase is concluded by completing the worksheet, upon which you will identify some triggers that you will likely be confronting over the next period of time (e.g., one week). Extra copies of the worksheet can be copied so that you can work toward self-regulation, intentionality, and narrative construction on several "reactive behaviors" simultaneously. It is also suggested that you maintain a journal in which you can record your thoughts, feelings, insights, and narratives as you navigate through the Pinnacle Program.

Phase III: Practice (Coaching and Desensitization)

The third phase of the Pinnacle Program is also the least structured. For many clients, this phase and subsequent sessions will look more like performance coaching than therapy. It will simply involve more of what has already been done – helping them identify triggers, encouraging them to practice self-regulation, and helping them to make good sense of how their past experiences have resulted in perceived threats in the present. In addition, we will want to make ample opportunity for them to share their narratives of trauma, pain, and fear and support whatever affect comes with these narratives. For clients who have minimal to moderate levels of posttraumatic stress, this version of the Pinnacle Program is often sufficient. They are frequently ready to terminate therapy with satisfaction in 6–12 sessions.

For those participants who are employing the Pinnacle Program in a self-help model, this phase involves the continuing practice of confronting triggers with relaxed bodies and regular meetings with your partner/coach/mentor to report progress, share narratives, and address problems. This third phase works well in a small group format (5–8 participants) of 60–90 minutes, during which each participant can take a turn to discuss successes and challenges they encountered during the intersession between group meetings. The support and identification participants experience in a group format is even more potent than individual meetings with a partner.

This phase of participation in the Pinnacle Program, however, often takes on a different timbre for individuals who have significant levels of posttraumatic stress. They often find themselves – after successfully completing the first two phases of the Pinnacle Program – frustrated, angry, and sometimes hopeless that their progress in this third phase has not been more bountiful. It is important for the participant who encounters early "failure" with the Pinnacle Program to not give up. Often these early difficulties are simply pointing to a more intensive traumatic and traumatized past that will need some focused clinical work – usually of a short duration – before they find themselves becoming successful with the Pinnacle model.

For participants of the Pinnacle Programwho experience these setbacks in the third phase and are unable to negotiate the confrontation of triggers while keeping their bodies relaxed, and who find themselves continuing to act in ways that are breaches of their integrity, there is still much hope! If you are one of these people, then it is recommended that you consult a psychotherapist specializing in treating traumatic stress. It is even further recommended that you consult one who is trained in Eye Movement Desensitization and Reprocessing (see http://www.emdr.com/clinic.htm) and explain to them your work with the Pinnacle Program. If they are good trauma therapists who are trained in EMDR, they will immediately understand when you describe to them your difficulty remaining self-regulated while confronting triggers and will be able to help you to desensitize and reprocess your past traumatic memories sufficiently so that, following this successful brief treatment, you should find yourself able to successfully confront these triggers with a relaxed body and intentional behaviors. It is further recommended that you create a consulting relationship with this therapist, much like you would with a dentist or family doctor. You may decide that you want to desensitize and reprocess additional trauma memories with this therapist or you may decide to return to the self-directed practice of the Pinnacle Program. Either way is fine as long as you are not experiencing increased symptoms (e.g., sleep problems, anxiety, depression, suicidal thoughts, compulsive or impulsive behavior, etc.). If you are experiencing exacerbated symptoms of traumatic stress, you should continue to work with a therapist until you have become stabilized for at least 2–4 weeks.

As participants continue to practice the Pinnacle Program, they find themselves able to practice intentional living with increased simplicity – even though self-regulation continues to require ongoing "bodyful" awareness. It is at this juncture that participants begin to discover the ultimate simplicity of the Pinnacle Program that is summarized in the "Formula for Hope #2" in Figure 8.

Clinical Note:
Clinicians will need to utilize all their relational skills to reassure their clients that this is simply part of the process of healing and some brief additional therapeutic activities need to be completed before they will be able to enjoy the full benefits of their hard work. Helping them to make sense of why they are falling short of being able to remain self-regulated and intentional during the activities of their lives is valuable both for the client and for maintaining the therapeutic relationship. It is crucial to help clients gain the insight that they are being intruded upon by their trauma memories with such ferocity that they are becoming immediately overwhelmed, SNS dominant, and reactive. It is also the therapist's task to help them understand that this continued reactivity is not a moral failing on their part. It is, instead, a testament to the intensity of the "injury" they suffered, and continue to suffer, from the traumatic experiences of their past.

Using the worksheet, we can point to square 5 and explain to our clients that the intrusions from their past traumatic experiences are coming forward into present consciousness with such intensity ("lightning bolt" on the worksheet) that is preventing them from being able to practice self-regulation when they encounter certain triggers. We ask them to identify the triggers they have experienced during their recent past that produced reactive behaviors. We then explain to them that it is likely that these triggers represent a memory or group of memories that were traumatic or painful experiences. We further explain that their adaptation to these traumatic and painful experiences was to orient themselves to avoid anything in the future that reminded them of these experiences. Anytime they encountered a reminder, they perceived it as a threat, their SNS activated, and they frequently attempted to avoid contact with this reminder.

Intention into Words
+ RELAXATION

Comfort in Body
Increased Thinking Capacity
Ability to Live with Intentionality & Integrity

Figure 8. Formula for Hope #2

Work over the next few sessions will focus upon helping clients desensitize and reprocess the trauma memory(ies) associated with the trigger(s). The goal of this desensitization and reprocessing work is to diminish the intensity of the intrusions – the perceived threats – sufficiently so that our clients can begin to self-regulate and remain relaxed when confronting these triggers. In the Pinnacle Program, this is always the single goal of regressive desensitization and reprocessing work with clients. Therapists do not employ therapeutic skills to develop insight, trigger abreactions, or to change beliefs. While all these may occur as byproducts of this work, the goal remains only to desensitize and reprocess the memory sufficiently so that our clients can practice self-regulation without being overwhelmed in the present. Please review the current volume of *Trauma Practice: Tools for Stabilization & Recovery* for additional interventions. It is important that the clinician work with whatever method of desensitization they enjoy a sense of mastery of. Cognitive Behavioral Therapy (e.g., Direct Therapeutic Exposure, Dialectical Behavioral Therapy, Prolonged Exposure, Cognitive Processing Therapy, etc); Neuro-Linguistic Programming (NLP)/Hypnotic Methods; Traumatic Incident Reduction (TIR); Narrative Therapy; and the TRI Method all have been the subjects of published studies that report effectiveness with PTSD symptoms. Eye-Movement Desensitization and Reprocessing (EMDR), however, is the recommended method for this phase of treatment. The procedure and philosophy of EMDR fits perfectly with the Pinnacle Program. For those who are aware of the EMDR protocol, the "triggers" from the Pinnacle Program fit perfectly as the "target" for the EMDR setup. EMDR, better than the other methods mentioned above, facilitates the client to desensitize and reprocess multiple trauma memories that may be associated with a particular trigger inside a single session. The other methods, which each have their value, require that each trauma memory be addressed individually. The use of one of these other models may require a longer treatment trajectory to achieve sufficient desensitization.

Clients who are able to successfully desensitize and reprocess a set of trauma memories and find that they are now able to effectively relax their bodies in the context of triggers that had previously been overwhelming often gain a renewed sense of hope and commitment to therapy. As they experience themselves successfully maintaining intentionality, where they previously capitulated to their fear, clients begin to believe that they just might be able to find a life that is no longer based in fear, pain, avoidance, and despair. They begin to see the possibility of living a life of principle-based intention and a pathway to a future where, truly, anything is possible for them. Lost dreams awaken.

Conclusion

The Pinnacle Program has provided relief from chronic fear, anxiety, obsessive thoughts, compulsive behavior, traumatic stress, and depression for scores of clients and hundreds of workshop participants. While there is not yet published research on the effectiveness of the Pinnacle Program, it is built upon and around protocols and principles of CBT that have demonstrated effectiveness for treating anxiety, depression, and traumatic stress. Although this program is not offered here as a substitute for traditional therapeutic approaches, it is, however, offered as a framework within which an individual can augment and accelerate traditional approaches to psychotherapy by living lives of intention. For some, the Pinnacle Program will allow them to make significant gains in symptom reduction and intentional living with minimal needs for traditional psychotherapy. The main difference between this program and psychotherapy is that the goal of the Pinnacle Program is to help clients live an intentional, principle-based life in alliance with their own personal morality. The goal of traditional psychotherapy is symptom reduction. As I have attempted to demonstrate in this writing, the Pinnacle Program may accomplish this symptom reduction as a byproduct instead of the goal. This shift in focus and process produces a significantly different "feel" to psychotherapy and self-help. Instead of the allopathic model in which the therapist is the "doctor" who brings healing to patient; in the Pinnacle Program the therapist/helper is more of a "midwife" who supports the process of natural healing while assisting the client in removing the impediments to their own maturational trajectory.

In this self-help version of the Pinnacle Program, the participant selects his or her own partner/coach/mentor for this process. The Pinnacle Program will help individuals establish a pathway toward intentional living to begin to become the people they have always wanted to be, living the way they want to live, regardless of their history or present-day situations. The Pinnacle Program may provide a pathway of healing for some individuals that will allow them to completely circumvent traditional psychotherapy. Others may need a little help from a caring professional throughout their process.

As a self-help model, the Pinnacle Program is poised to become the first of its kind to show effectiveness in treating the symptoms of traumatic stress, anxiety, and depression. No self-help models have been discovered to demonstrate effectiveness with significantly lowering the symptoms traumatic stress in the literature reviewed for this article. It will be interesting to see whether the Pinnacle Program will be able to provide this lessening. I have watched countless clients lower their symptoms and, much more importantly, begin to live principle-based lives with which they are satisfied through practicing the simple principles of this program. I have received literally hundreds of emails from workshop participants who, after one day of training, have told me that their lives have transformed as a result of implementing these principles and practices. Currently, the Pinnacle Program as both an adjunct to psychotherapy and as a self-help protocol is experimental. I am unable to make any scientific claims as to its effectiveness or to its safety – although it is difficult to see how it could be harmful. I am in the process of beginning research on this model and only time and careful data collection will be able to demonstrate conclusively whether the Pinnacle Model is effective either for symptom reduction or in facilitating intentional living, leading individuals to greater satisfaction with their lives. I do, however, expect that positive results will follow. You are invited to conduct your own research. If you find the practice of the principles and exercises of the Pinnacle Program helpful, then continue to utilize this program, free of charge, for as long as you find it helpful. If you do not find it useful, you have lost precious little in your attempts. If you do choose to apply the Pinnacle Program to your life, I would appreciate hearing from you, whether the program has been helpful or not. My contact information appears at the end of this article.

The single most exciting thing about the Pinnacle Program, for me, is its immediacy for hope. The ability to show clients how, within a single session, they can move away from years of suffering with the symptoms of traumatic stress and anxiety brought on by the chronic dominance of the SNS into the comfort and intentionality of parasympathetic dominance is frequently staggering for both the client and the clinician. To witness the dawn of hope upon the faces and in the hearts of those suffering survivors who sit across from me and for whom there has been no hope, sometimes for decades, count among the greatest experiences of my lifetime. Since beginning to employ the principles of the Pinnacle Program, this has become an ever more frequent occurrence.

If there is any way that I can assist a reader of this article in helping to implement the Pinnacle Program in their lives or the lives of others, I welcome your contact.

J. Eric Gentry, PhD

2. Compassion Fatigue: The Crucible of Transformation

Introduction

In this book, we formulate a process to assist therapists to guide their clients from trauma to recovery. However, no book on this topic can be complete without a section on care for the care provider. We understand that those who choose this field have chosen to bear witness to the plight of trauma survivors. In the course of this meaningful work there remains the ever-present possibility of encountering wounds so shattering that the impact creates a secondary wound for the helper.

Most of us receiving professional training were never fortunate enough to receive a clear and compassionate message that there may be a cost to our caring work. Instead we have experienced the pain of our work and then the additional wound of being shamed and blamed by colleagues, supervisors, and the very system that trained us professionally. We hope to send a new message: one of hope, caring, and resiliency. If you find yourself struggling with the impact of your work, know that there is hope and a road to recovery. Just as you provide nurturing care to your clients, know there is also care available for you.

The following text first appeared in *The Journal of Trauma Practice* in 2002 and is presented here, with permission, in its entirety. It was provided by J. Eric Gentry to provide a clear message that caregivers never have to feel shame, blame, or guilt if they are impacted by their caring work.

Compassion Fatigue: The Crucible of Transformation[1]

On October 19, 2001 I co-facilitated a Critical Incident Stress Debriefing (CISD; Mitchell, 1995) in New York City for 12 mid-level retail managers who had been working two blocks from the World Trade Center on September 11, 2001. As this group navigated through the CISD and its cognitive – affective – cognitive "schwoop" (Norman, 2001), that hallmark of emergency psychology, one person began to describe the debris falling from the crumbling towers by saying, "in my mind I see chunks of concrete falling from the building but I know it was really people that I saw falling ... jumping." As she spoke, I could not help myself from forming my own images of falling debris coalescing into anatomical features. Another participant reported that the worst part of September 11 for him was the emergence of recurrent intrusive images and nightmares. However, the intrusions he was experiencing were not of the horrors he saw in lower Manhattan; instead they were of tracer rounds from automatic rifles firing over his and his mother's head when he was a child fleeing Vietnam in 1975. As he described the spontaneous emergence of these memories, brought to consciousness for the first time in 26 years, I began to recall images from some of the hundreds of combat trauma narratives I have heard from the number of combat veterans that I have treated. I also began to feel some anxiety for the co-facilitator who was leading this debriefing, as this was his 30th straight day of providing trauma relief services in New York City and he was a Vietnam combat veteran.

While participating in this debriefing, I was acutely aware of my powerlessness to prevent the images, thoughts, and feelings shared by the participants from finding their way into parallel associations in my own consciousness. Having spent the past five years studying and treating compassion fatigue, I knew that I was at high risk for the development of secondary traumatic

---

[1] This text first appeared as an article by J. Eric Gentry in *The Journal of Trauma Practice,* 1(3–4), 37–61. © 2002 The Haworth Press, Binghampton, NY, USA. Article copies are available from The Haworth Document Delivery Service: 1-800-HAWORTH, e-mail: docdelivery@haworthpress.com.

stress symptoms. For the next several weeks I experienced recurrent images and accompanying arousal from this and other experiences in New York. It was only after extensive support from colleagues and my work, as a client, with Eye Movement Desensitization and Reprocessing (EMDR, Shapiro, 1995), that I was able to relegate these images and feelings from the encroaching present into the near-distant past.

Thousands of emergency service and mental health professionals have labored heroically to assist survivors of the events of 9/11/01. These service professionals have witnessed events and heard stories of incredible courage and resiliency in the course of providing assistance to the survivors. They have also been exposed to incidents and reports of life-shattering pain, terror, and loss. There is no doubt that there are great rewards associated with providing care and assistance to survivors of trauma; for those of us who have chosen traumatology as a professional path, there is no sweeter experience than witnessing a survivor emerge transformed and fortified from the dark jungle of posttraumatic symptoms. There is also, however, little doubt that serving these survivors exacts a toll that while minimal for some caregivers, can be devastating for others. As Viktor Frankl, one of the twentieth century's greatest traumatologists, simultaneously warns and encourages: "That which is to give light must endure burning" (Frankl, 1963, p. 129).

This chapter explores the potential causes, prevention, and treatments of compassion fatigue (Figley, 1995), the deleterious effects of helping the traumatized, as it relates to the tragedy of September 11, 2001. It is offered with the hope that it may help some of those dedicated to being of service to trauma survivors, in any context, to continue being givers of light, burning ever more brightly, and never burning out.

Compassion Fatigue

The notion that working with people in pain extracts a significant cost from the caregiver is not new. Although the costs vary and have been lamented from time immemorial, anyone who has sat at the bedside of a seriously ill or recently bereaved loved one knows the toll involved in devoting singular attention to the needs of another suffering person. Only in recent years, however, has there been a substantial effort to examine the effects on the caregiver of bearing witness to the indescribable wounds inflicted by traumatic experiences. The exploration and examination of these effects evolved throughout the last century and comes to us from a wide variety of sources.

One of the first earliest references in the scientific literature regarding this cost of caring comes from Carl G. Jung in The Psychology of Dementia Praecox (Jung, 1907). In this text, Jung discusses the challenges of countertransference – the therapist's conscious and unconscious reactions to the patient in the therapeutic situation – and the particular counter-transference difficulties analysts encounter when working with psychotic patients. He boldly prescribes a treatment stance in which the therapist participates in the delusional fantasies and hallucinations with the patient. Nevertheless, he warns that this participation in the patient's darkly painful fantasy world of traumatic images has significant deleterious effects for the therapist, especially the neophyte and/or the therapist who has not resolved his/her own developmental and traumatic issues (Sedgewick, 1995).

The study of countertransference produced the first writings in the field of psychotherapy that systematically explored the effects of psychotherapy upon the therapist (Haley, 1974; Danieli, 1982; Lindy, 1988; Wilson & Lindy, 1994; Karakashian, 1994; Pearlman & Saakvitne, 1995). Recent texts have suggested that therapists sometimes experience countertransference reactions that imitate the symptoms of their clients (Herman, 1992; Pearlman & Saakvitne, 1995). For instance, when working with survivors of traumatic experiences, authors have reported countertransference phenomena that mimic the symptoms of post-traumatic stress disorder (PTSD; Lindy, 1988; Wilson & Lindy, 1994; Pearlman & Saakvitne, 1995).

Business and industry, with their progressive focus upon productivity in the last half of the twentieth century, have provided us with the concept of burnout (Freudenberger, 1974; Maslach, 1976, 1982) to describe the deleterious effects the environmental demands of the workplace have on the worker. Burnout, or "the syndrome of emotional exhaustion, depersonalization, and reduced personal accomplishment" (Maslach, 1976, p. 56), has been used to describe the chronic effects that psychotherapists suffer as a result of interactions with their clients and/or the demands of their workplace (Freudenberger, 1974; Cherniss, 1980; Farber, 1983; Sussman, 1992; Grosch & Olsen, 1994; Maslach & Goldberg, 1998). Research has shown that therapists are particularly vulnerable to burnout because of personal isolation, ambiguous successes and the emotional drain of remaining empathetic (McCann & Pearlman, 1990). Moreover, burnout not only is psychologically debilitating to therapists, but also impairs the therapist's capacity to deliver competent mental health services (Farber, 1983). The literature on burnout, with its twenty-five year history, thoroughly describes the phenomena and prescribes preventive and treatment interventions for helping professionals.

The study of the effects of trauma has also promoted a better understanding of the negative effects of helping. Psychological reactions to trauma have been described over the past one hundred and fifty years by various names such as "shell shock", "combat neurosis", "railroad spine", and "combat fatigue" (Shalev, Bonne, & Eth, 1996). However, not until 1980 was the latest designation for these reactions, posttraumatic stress disorder (PTSD), formally recognized as an anxiety disorder in the Diagnostic and Statistical Manual of Mental Disorders-III (DSM-III, American Psychiatric Association, 1980; Matsakis, 1994). Since that time, research into posttraumatic stress has grown at an exponential rate (Figley, 1995; Wilson & Lindy, 1994) and the field of traumatology has been established with two of its own journals, several professional organizations, and unique professional identity (Figley, 1988; Bloom, 2000; Gold & Faust, 2001).

As therapists are increasingly called upon to assist survivors of violent crime, natural disasters, childhood abuse, torture, acts of genocide, political persecution, war, and now terrorism (Sexton, 1999), discussion regarding the reactions of therapists and other helpers to working with trauma survivors has recently emerged in the traumatology literature (Figley, 1983, 1995; Danieli, 1988; McCann & Pearlman, 1990; Pearlman & Saakvitne, 1995; Stamm, 1995). Professionals who listen to reports of trauma, horror, human cruelty and extreme loss can become overwhelmed and may begin to experience feelings of fear, pain and suffering similar to that of their clients. They may also experience PTSD symptoms similar to their clients', such as intrusive thoughts, nightmares, avoidance and arousal, as well as changes in their relationships to their selves, their families, friends and communities (Figley, 1995; McCann & Pearlman, 1990, Salston, 1999). Therefore, they may themselves come to need assistance to cope with the effects of listening to others' traumatic experiences (Figley, 1995; Pearlman & Saakvitne, 1995; Saakvitne, 1996; Gentry, Baranowsky, & Dunning, 2002).

While the empirical literature has been slow to develop in this area, there is an emerging body of scientific publications that attempt to identify and define the traumatization of helpers through their efforts of helping. Pearlman and Saakvitne (1995), Figley (1995), and Stamm (1995) all authored and/or edited texts that explored this phenomenon among helping professionals during the same pivotal year. The terms "vicarious traumatization" (McCann & Pearlman, 1990; Pearlman & Saakvitne, 1995), "secondary traumatic stress" (Figley, 1987; Stamm, 1995) and "compassion fatigue" (Figley, 1995) have all become cornerstones in the vernacular of describing the deleterious effects that helpers suffer when working with trauma survivors.

Vicarious traumatization (McCann & Pearlman, 1990) refers to the transmission of traumatic stress through observation and/or hearing others' stories of traumatic events and the resultant shift/distortions that occur in the caregiver's perceptual and meaning systems. Secondary traumatic stress occurs when one is exposed to extreme events directly experienced by another and becomes overwhelmed by this secondary exposure to trauma (Figley & Kleber, 1995). Several theories have been offered but none has been able to conclusively demonstrate the mechanism that accounts for the transmission of traumatic stress from one individual to another. It has been hypothesized that the caregiver's level of empathy with the traumatized individual plays a significant role in this transmission (Figley, 1995) and some budding empirical data to support this hypothesis (Salston, 2000).

Figley (1995) also proposes that the combined effects of the caregiver's continuous visualizing of clients' traumatic images added to the effects of burnout can create a condition progressively debilitating the caregiver that he has called "compassion stress." This construct holds that exposure to clients' stories of traumatization can produce a form of posttraumatic stress disorder in which Criterion A, or "the event" criterion, is met through listening to, instead of the in vivo experiencing of, a traumatic event. The symptoms of compassion fatigue, divided into categories of intrusive, avoidance, and arousal symptoms, are summarized in Table 1.

As a result of our work with hundreds of caregivers suffering the effects of compassion fatigue, we have augmented Figley's (1995) definition to include preexisting and/or concomitant primary posttraumatic stress and its symptoms. Many caregivers, especially those providing on-site services, will have had firsthand exposure to the traumatic event(s) to which they are responding (Pole et al., 2001; Marmar et al., 1999). For many, these symptoms of PTSD will have a delayed onset and not become manifest until some time later. We have also found that many caregivers enter the service field with a host of traumatic experiences in their developmental past (Gentry, 1999). There may have been no symptoms associated with these events, or the symptoms related to them may have remained sub-clinical. However, we have observed that as these caregivers begin to encounter the traumatic material presented by clients, many of them begin to develop clinical PTSD symptoms associated with their previously "benign" historical experiences.

In our efforts to treat compassion fatigue, we have concluded that it is often necessary to successfully address and resolve primary traumatic stress before addressing any issues of secondary traumatic stress and/or burnout. Additionally, we have discerned an interactive, or

Table 1. Preferred psychotherapy techniques for different PTSD target symptoms		
Intrusive symptoms	**Avoidance symptoms**	**Arousal symptoms**
• Thoughts and images associated with client's traumatic experiences • Obsessive and compulsive desire to help certain clients • Client/work issues encroaching upon personal time • Inability to "let go" of work-related matters • Perception of survivors as fragile and needing the assistance of caregiver ("savior") • Thoughts and feelings of inadequacy as a caregiver Sense of entitlement or specialness • Perception of the world in terms of victims and perpetrators • Personal activities interrupted by work-related issues	• Silencing Response (avoiding hearing/witnessing client's traumatic material) • Loss of enjoyment in activities/cessation of self care activities • Loss of energy • Loss of hope/sense of dread working with certain clients • Loss of sense of competence/potency • Isolation • Secretive self-medication/addiction (alcohol, drugs, work, sex, food, spending, etc) • Relational dysfunction	• Increased anxiety • Impulsivity/reactivity • Increased perception of demand/threat (in both job and environment) • Increased frustration/anger • Sleep disturbance • Difficulty concentrating • Change in weight/appetite • Somatic symptoms

synergistic, effect among primary traumatic stress, secondary traumatic stress, and burnout symptoms in the life of an afflicted caregiver. Experiencing symptoms from any one of these three sources appears to diminish resiliency and lower thresholds for the adverse impact of the other two. This seems to lead to a rapid onset of severe symptoms that can become extremely debilitating to the caregiver within a very short period of time.

Accelerated Recovery Program for Compassion Fatigue

In 1997, two Green Cross Scholars and one doctoral student under the direction and supervision of Charles Figley at Florida State University developed the Accelerated Recovery Program for Compassion Fatigue (Gentry, Baranowsky, & Dunning, 2002; Gentry & Baranowsky, 1998, 1999, 1999a, 1999b). This five-session manualized and copyrighted protocol[2] was designed to address the symptoms of secondary traumatic stress and burnout, or compassion fatigue, in caregivers. Phase one clinical trials with this protocol werecompleted with the developers and seven volunteers from various disciplines and backgrounds who had experience working with trauma survivors.[3] The qualitative data obtained from these initial volunteers were utilized to create the final version of the protocol. Each of these participants reported clinically significant lessening of compassion fatigue symptoms with one exception.[4]

The Accelerated Recovery Program (ARP) was presented in the fall of 1997 at the International Society for Traumatic Stress Studies (ISTSS) in Montreal, Canada. In attendance at this presentation was an official with the Federal Bureau of Investigation who requested that the developers provide training to his staff, and, subsequent to this training, the Accelerated Recovery Program was adopted for use in this agency (McNally, 1998, personal communication). As a result of contacts made through the FBI, twelve professional helpers who have provided ongoing assistance to the survivors of the bombing of the Murrah Building in Oklahoma City requested treatment for their compassion fatigue symptoms through the Traumatology Institute at Florida State University. The ARP provided statistically and clinically significant successful treatment for each of these professionals (Gentry, 2000). Subsequent presentations on the ARP at ISTSS meetings in 1998, 1999, and the development of the Compassion Fatigue Specialist Training (CFST) have lead to the successful treatment of hundreds of caregivers with compassion fatigue symptoms through the Accelerated Recovery Program all over the world. This program is now available online at www.ticlearn.com.

Compassion Fatigue Specialist Training: Training-as-Treatment

In late 1998, Gentry and Baranowsky, two of the developers of the Accelerated Recovery Program, were approached by the Traumatology Institute at Florida State University to create a training program for helping professionals interested in developing expertise in treating compassion fatigue. Through initial consultations, it was decided that the training would be designed around the ARP Model and that the participants would receive training on the implementation of the five sessions of this protocol. In addition, the training was designed to provide the participants with an in-depth understanding of the etiology, phenomenology and treatment/prevention of compassion fatigue, including secondary traumatic stress and burnout. The participants of this training would be recognized by Florida State Universitys Trau-

---

2 *Compassion Fatigue Treatment Manual (ARP)* (Gentry & Baranowsky, 1998) available from Psych Ink Resources, 45 Sheppard Ave., Suite 419 Toronto, Ontario, Canada, M2N 5W9 or http://www.psychink.com.

3 These trials were completed with volunteers who were marriage & family therapists, a trauma therapist from South Africa, and a volunteer who had been providing relief work in Sarajevo.

4 This participant uncovered a primary traumatic experience for which she was previously amnestic. She left the country before her primary or secondary trauma could be successfully addressed and resolved.

matology Institute as Compassion Fatigue Specialists and authorized to implement the Accelerated Recovery Program for other caregivers suffering from compassion fatigue symptoms.

In their design of the program, the developers decided that the participants should receive first-hand experiential training for each of the interventions used in the Accelerated Recovery Program. With this in mind, the 17-hour training was developed and manualized (Gentry & Baranowsky, 1998, 1999a, 1999b) with a focus upon the experiential components of the ARP. This phase in development of the Compassion Fatigue Specialist Training (CFST) was the first conceptualization of the "training-as-treatment" (Gentry, 2000) model for addressing the participants' symptoms of compassion fatigue. The rationale was that since the interventions of the ARP were effective working with individuals, the interventions would also be effective with these symptoms, albeit to a lesser degree, with the participants of the training.

It was then decided that the collection of baseline and outcome data would be conducted from the first training that was implemented in January of 1999. Baseline and post-training scores from compassion fatigue, compassion satisfaction, and burnout sub-scales of the Compassion Satisfaction/Fatigue Self-Test (Figley, 1995; Figley & Stamm, 1996) were collected. Data were analyzed for 166 participants who successfully completed the CFS Training between January 1999 and January 2001 (Gentry, 2000). The protocol demonstrated clinically and statically significant results ($p < .001$) when pretraining and posttraining scores on the compassion fatigue, compassion satisfaction, and burnout subscales of the Compassion Satisfaction/Fatigue Self-Test (Figley & Stamm, 1996) were compared.

Treatment and Prevention: Active Ingredients

It has been demonstrated that the potential to develop negative symptoms associated with our work in providing services to trauma survivors, especially the symptoms of secondary traumatic stress, increases as our exposure to their traumatic material increases (McCann & Pearlman, 1990; Salston, 2000). We believe that no one who chooses to work with trauma survivors is immune to the potential deleterious effects of this work. However, in our work with providing effective treatment to hundreds of caregivers with compassion fatigue symptoms, either individually through the ARP or in CFS training groups, we have identified some enduring principles, techniques, and ingredients that seem to consistently lead to these positive treatment outcomes and enhanced resiliency.

Intentionality

Initiation of effective resolution of compassion fatigue symptoms requires specific recognition and acceptance of the symptoms and their causes by the caregiver, along with a decision to address and resolve these symptoms. Many caregivers who experience symptoms of compassion fatigue will attempt to ignore their distress until a threshold of discomfort is reached. For many caregivers this may mean that they are unable to perform their jobs as well as they once did or as well as they would like due to the symptoms they are experiencing. For others, it may entail the progressive debilitation associated with somatic symptoms or the embarrassment and pain associated with secretive self-destructive comfort-seeking behaviors. Whatever the impetus, we have found that successful amelioration of compassion fatigue symptoms requires that the caregiver intentionally acknowledge and address, rather than avoid, these symptoms and their causes. Additionally, we have found the use of goal-setting and the development of a personal/professional mission statement to be invaluable in moving away from the reactivity associated with the victimization of compassion fatigue and toward the resiliency and intentionality of mature caregiving.

Connection

One of the ways trauma seems to affect us all, caregivers included, is to leave us with a sense of disconnected isolation. A common thread we have found with sufferers of compassion fatigue symptoms has been the progressive loss in their sense of connection and community. Many caregivers become increasingly isolated as their symptoms intensify. Fear of being perceived as weak, impaired, or incompetent by peers and clients, along with time constraints and loss of interest, have all been cited by caregivers suffering from compassion fatigue as reasons for diminished intimate and collegial connection. The development and maintenance of healthy relationships, which the caregiver uses for both support and to share/dilute the images and stories associated with secondary traumatic stress, may become a powerful mitigating factor in resolving and preventing compassion fatigue symptoms. Often the bridge for this connection is established in the peer-to-peer offering of the ARP, during which the facilitator works intentionally to develop a strong relationship with the caregiver suffering compassion fatigue symptoms.

In the CFST, we facilitate exercises specifically designed to dismantle interpersonal barriers and enhance self-disclosure. It seems that it is through these relational connections that the caregivers suffering compassion fatigue are able to gain insight and understanding that their symptoms are not an indication of some pathological weakness or disease, but are instead natural consequences of providing care for traumatized individuals. In addition, with the enhanced self-acceptance attained through self-disclosure with and by empathetic and understanding peers, caregivers are able to begin to see their symptoms as indicators of the developmental changes needed in both their self-care and caregiving practices. We have seen that a warm, supportive environment in which caregivers are able to discuss intrusive traumatic material, difficult clients, symptoms, fears, shame, and secrets with peers to be one of the most critical ingredients in the resolution and continued prevention of compassion fatigue.

Anxiety Management/Self-Soothing

It is our belief that providing caregiving services while experiencing intense anxiety is one of the primary means by which compassion fatigue symptoms are contracted and exacerbated. Alternately stated, to the degree that a caregiver is able to remain non-anxious (relaxed pelvic floor muscles), we believe, s/he will maintain resistance to the development of symptoms of compassion fatigue. The ability to self-regulate and soothe anxiety and stress is thought to be a hallmark of maturity. The mastery of these skills comes only with years of practice. However, if we fail to develop the capacity for self-regulation, if we are unable to internally attenuate our own levels of arousal, then we are susceptible to perceiving as threats those people, objects, and situations to which we respond with anxiety – believing that benign people, objects, and situations are dangerous. As one very insightful and astute psychologist who was a participant in the CFST stated "Maybe the symptoms of compassion fatigue are a good thing, they force us to become stronger." It does seem to be true that those caregivers with well-developed self-regulation skills who do not resort to self-destructive and addictive comfort-seeking behaviors are unlikely to suffer symptoms of compassion fatigue.

In both the ARP and the CFST, we work rigorously with participant caregivers to help them develop self-management plans that will assist them in achieving and maintaining an in vivo nonanxious presence. This nonanxious presence extends far beyond a calm outward appearance. Instead, it entails the ability to maintain a level of relaxed mindfulness and comfort in one's own body. This ability to remain non-anxious when confronted with the pain, horror, loss, and powerlessness associated with the traumatic experiences in the lives of clients, of having the capacity to calmly "bear witness," remains a key ingredient in the resolution and prevention of compassion fatigue symptoms.

Self-Care

Closely associated with self-management is the concept of self-care, or the ability to refill and refuel oneself in healthy ways. It is quite common for caregivers to find themselves anxious during and after working with severely traumatized individuals. Instead of developing a system of healthy practices for resolving this anxiety – such as sharing with colleagues, exercise, meditation, nutrition, and spirituality – many caregivers find themselves redoubling their work efforts. Frequently this constricting cycle of working harder in an attempt to feel better creates a distorted sense of entitlement that can lead to a breach of personal and professional boundaries. We have worked with many caregivers who have reported falling prey to compulsive behaviors such as overeating, overspending, or alcohol/drug abuse in an effort to soothe the anxiety they feel from the perceived demands of their work. Others with whom we have worked have self-consciously admitted to breaching professional boundaries and ethics when at the low point in this cycle, distortedly believing that they "deserve" this "special" treatment or reward.

Meta-analyses of psychotherapy outcomes consistently point toward the quality of the relationship between therapist and client as the single most important ingredient in positive outcomes (Bergin & Garfield, 1994). The integrity and quality of this relationship is contingent upon the therapist's maintenance of his/her instrument, the "self of the therapist." When caregivers fail to maintain a life that is rich with meaning and gratification outside the professional arena, then they often look to work as the sole source of these commodities. In this scenario, caregivers interact with their clients from a stance of depletion and need. It is completely understandable that this orientation would produce symptoms in caregivers. Conversely, professionals who responsibly pursue and acquire this sense of aliveness outside the closed system of their professional role are able to engage in work with traumatized individuals while sharing their own fullness, meaning, and joy. The cycle of depletion by our work and intentionally refilling ourselves in our lives outside of work, often on a daily basis, may have been what Frankl meant when he challenged us to "endure burning."

One of the most important aspects of this category of self-care that we have found in our work with caregivers has been the development and maintenance of a regular exercise regimen. No other single behavior seems to be as important as regular aerobic and anaerobic activity. In addition to exercise, good nutrition, artistic expression/discipline (e.g., piano lessons and composition, dance classes and choreography, structural planning and building), meditation/mindfulness, outdoor recreation, and spirituality all seem to be important ingredients to a good self-care plan.

We have found a few caregivers with compassion fatigue symptoms that seemed to be at least partially caused by working beyond their level of skill. Working with traumatized individuals, families, and communities is a highly skilled activity that demands many years of training in many different areas before one gains a sense of mastery. Trying to shortcut this process by prematurely working with trauma survivors without adequate training and supervision can very easily overwhelm even seasoned clinicians, much less neophytes. While empirical research has not yet addressed the effects of working beyond levels of competency or of providing services while impaired with stress symptoms has upon the care provider, especially in contexts of mass casualties like we have witnessed in New York City, we believe that these factors contribute significantly to the frequency, duration and intensity of compassion fatigue symptoms.

Sometimes training in the area of treating trauma, especially experiential trainings such as EMDR (Shapiro, 1995) or TIR (French & Harris, 1998), can have a powerful ameliorative effect upon compassion fatigue, bringing a sense of empowerment to a caregiver who was previously overwhelmed. The caveat here is that there exists some danger that an overwhelmed therapist who has been recently trained in one of these powerful techniques may emerge from the training with an inflated sense of skill and potency. Newly empowered, this therapist may be tempted to practice even further beyond their level of competence and skill. This scenario highlights the importance of good professional supervision during the developmental phases of a traumatologist's career. In addition, many therapists working with trauma survivors have found it helpful to receive periodic "checkups" with a trusted professional or peer supervisor. This is especially true during and immediately following deployment in a disaster or critical incident situation. These professional and peer supervisory relationships can serve as excellent opportunities to share, and therefore dilute the effects, or the artifacts of secondary traumatic stress that may have been collected while in service to trauma survivors. Professional supervision is also reported to have an overall ameliorative effect upon compassion fatigue symptoms (Pearlman, 1995; Catherall, 1995).

Every caregiver's self-care needs are different. Some will need to remain vigilant in the monitoring and execution of their self-care plan, while others will, seemingly, be able to maintain resiliency with minimal effort. However, we strongly urge the caregiver who specializes in work with trauma and trauma survivors to develop a comprehensive self-care plan that addresses and meets the caregiver's individual needs for each of the areas discussed in this article. With this self-care plan in place, the caregiver can now practice with the assurance that they are maximizing resiliency toward and prevention of the symptoms of compassion fatigue that is akin to the protection of wearing a seatbelt while driving an automobile.

It should be noted that those care providers responding on-site to crisis situations, such as those caused by the events of September 11, may be limited in their ability to employ habitual self-care activities. They may not have access to gymnasiums or exercise facilities, nutritious food and water may be scarce for a period of time, and it is doubtful that care providers deployed in situations of mass destruction will have access to their traditional support network. While most trauma responders are a hardy and resilient breed, we simply cannot sustain the rigors of this depleting and intensive work without intentional concern for our own health and welfare. Making the best use of available resources to establish respite and sanctuary for ourselves, even in the most abject of circumstances, can have an enormous effect in minimizing our symptoms and maximizing our sustained effectiveness. Many responders have reported acts of kindness as simple as the gift of a bottle of water, a pat on the back, or an opportunity to share a meal with another responder as having a powerfully positive impact upon their morale and energy during these difficult times.

Narrative

Many researchers and writers have identified the creation of a chronological verbal and/or graphic narrative as an important ingredient in the healing of traumatic stress, especially intrusive symptoms (Tinnin, 1994; van der Kolk, McFarlane, & Weisaeth 1996; Foa et al., 1999). We have found that a creation of a time-line narrative of a caregiving career that identifies the experiences and the clients from which the caregiver developed primary and secondary traumatic stress is invaluable in the resolution of compassion fatigue symptoms, especially those associated with secondary traumatic stress. In the ARP, we instruct the participant/caregiver to "tell your story ... from the beginning – the first experiences in your life that led you toward caregiving – to the present." We use a video camera to record this narrative and ask the caregiver to watch it later that same day. They are to take care to identify the experiences that have led to any primary and secondary traumatic stress (intrusive symptoms) by constructing a graphic timeline. In the CFST, we utilize dyads in which two participants each take a one-hour block of time to verbalize their narrative while the other practices nonanxious "bearing witness" of this narrative.

Desensitization and Reprocessing

With the narrative completed and the identification of historical experiences resulting in primary and secondary traumatic stress, the caregiver is now ready to resolve these memories. In the ARP, we have utilized Eye Movement Dissociation and Reprocessing (Shapiro, 1989, 1995) as the method of choice for this work. In the CCFST, we utilize a hybridized version of a Neuro-Linguistic Programming Anchoring Technique (Baranowsky & Gentry, 1998a, 1998b). Any method that simultaneously employs exposure and relaxation (i.e., reciprocal inhibition) is appropriate for this important cornerstone of treatment. We have had success utilizing Traumatic Incident Reduction (French & Harris, 1998), the anamnesis procedure from the Trauma Recovery Institute (TRI) Method (Tinnin, 1994), or many of the techniques from Cognitive-Behavioral Therapy (see this text; Foa & Meadows, 1997; Follette, Ruzek, & Abueg, 1998; Rothbaum, Meadows, Resick, & Foy, 2000). With the successful desensitization and reprocessing of the caregiver's primary and secondary traumatic stress, and the cessation of intrusive symptoms, often comes a concomitant sense of rebirth, joy, and transformation. This important step and ingredient in the treatment of compassion fatigue should not be minimized or overlooked.

In our work with the responders of the Oklahoma City bombing, none reported experiencing intrusive symptoms of secondary and/or primary traumatic stress until several days, weeks, months, and sometimes years after their work at the site. From personal communication with an Incident Commander for a team of mental health responders who worked with over 2700 victims in New York City the first month after the attacks (Norman, personal communication, 2002), he indicated that at least one Compassion Fatigue Specialist was available to provide daily debriefing services for every ten (10) responders. He further indicated that if a responder began to report symptoms or show signs of significant traumatic stress they were provided with acute stabilization services by the team and arrangements were made for transportation back home with a referral to a mental health practitioner in the worker's home town. With the intense demands of critical incident work and the paramount importance of worker safety, attempts of desensitization and reprocessing care provider's primary and secondary traumatic stress while on-site seems counterproductive as it draws from the already depleted resources of the intervention team. For this reason, it is recommended that the worker engage in resolving the effects of accumulated traumatic memories only after safely returning to the existing resources and support offered by their family, friends, churches/synagogues, and health care professionals in their hometown.

Self-Supervision

This aspect of treatment is focused upon the correction of distorted and coercive cognitive styles. Distorted thinking may be developmental (i.e., existent prior to a caregiver's career), or may have been developed in response to primary and secondary traumatic stress later in life. Whatever the cause, we have found that once a caregiver contracts the negative symptoms of compassion fatigue, these symptoms will not fully resolve until distorted beliefs about self and the world are in the process of correction. This is especially true for the ways in which we supervise and motivate ourselves. Caregivers recovering from the symptoms of compassion fatigue will need to soften their critical and coercive self-talk and shift their motivational styles toward more self-accepting and affirming language and tone if they wish to resolve their compassion fatigue symptoms. For many this is a difficult, tedious, and painstaking breaking-of-bad-habits process than can take years to complete.

In the ARP and the CFST, we have employed an elegant and powerful technique called "video-dialogue" (Holmes & Tinnin, 1995) that accelerates this process significantly. This technique, adapted for use with the ARP, challenges the participant to write a letter to themselves from the perspective of a "Great Supervisor," lavishing upon themselves all the praise, support, and validation that they wish from others. They are then requested to read this letter into the eye of the camera. While watching back the videotape of this letter, the caregiver is asked to "pay attention to any negative or critical thought that thwarts your acceptance of this praise." Then, s/he is instructed to give these critical and negative thoughts a "voice," as these negative thoughts are articulated into the video camera, directed at the caregiver. This back-and-forth argument between the "self" and the "critical voice" of the caregiver continues on videotape until both "sides" begin to see the utility in both perspectives. With this completed, polarities relax, self-criticism softens, and integration is facilitated.

While this technique is powerfully evocative and can rapidly transform self-critical thinking styles, the Cognitive Therapy "triple column technique" (Burns, 1980), that helps identify particular cognitive distortions and challenges a client to rewrite these negative thoughts into ones that are more adaptive and satisfying will also work well for this task. Additionally, as caregivers suffering from compassion fatigue symptoms develop some mastery in resolving these internal polarities with themselves, they are challenged to identify and resolve polarities with significant others. Individuals traumatized from either primary or secondary sources who are able to "un-freeze" themselves from their polarities, resentments, conflicts, and cut-offs will be rewarded with less anxiety, a heightened sense of comfort inside their own skin, and a greater sense of freedom from the past to pursue their mission of the present and future.

The Crucible of Transformation

Our initial intent in developing the ARP was to simply gather a collection of powerful techniques and experiences that would rapidly ameliorate the suffering from symptoms of compassion fatigue in the lives of caregivers so that they would be able to return to their lives and their work refreshed and renewed. However, as we embarked upon yoking ourselves with the formidable task of sitting across from our peers who were suffering with these symptoms, many of whom were demoralized, hopeless, and desperate, we began to understand that recovery from compassion fatigue required significant changes in the foundational beliefs and lifestyles of the caregiver. As we navigated through the five sessions of the ARP with these suffering professionals we found that most underwent a significant transformation in the way in which they perceived their work and, ultimately, themselves.

Drawing from the work of David Schnarch (1991), who works with enmeshed couples to develop self-validated intimacy and achieve sexual potentials in their marriages, we began to see that many caregivers exhibited a similar form of enmeshment with their careers. We found that many of those suffering with compassion fatigue symptoms maintained an other-validated stance in their caregiving work – they were compelled to gain approval and feelings of worth from their clients, supervisors, and peers. In beginning to explore the developmental histories of many of the caregivers with whom we have worked, we found that many carried into their adult lives, and careers, unresolved attachment and developmental issues. For the caregiver who operates from an other-validated stance, clients, supervisors, and peers all represent potential threats when approval is withheld. These perceptions of danger and threat by the caregiver, which are enhanced by secondary traumatic stress contracted in work with trauma survivors, often lead to increased anxiety, feelings of victimization, and a sense of overwhelming powerlessness.

As the caregiver is able to evolve toward a more self-validated stance and become more grounded in the non-anxious present, these symptoms begin to permanently dissipate. Pearlman and Saakvitne (1995) urge therapists to "find self-worth that is not based on their professional achievements. It is essential to develop and nurture spiritual lives outside our work" (p. 396). While we have found no existing empirical data in this ripe area of study, from a treatment perspective we began to see how the symptoms of compassion fatigue make sense in the lives of many professional caregivers, urging them towards maturation.

Instead of viewing the symptoms of compassion fatigue as a pathological condition that requires some external treatment agent or techniques for resolution, we began to see these symptoms as indicators of the need for the professional caregiver to continue his/her development into matured caregiving and self-care styles and practices. From this perspective the symptoms of compassion fatigue can be interpreted as messages from what is right, good, and strong within us, rather than indicators of shameful weaknesses, defects, or sickness.

Through our continued work with caregivers suffering the effects of secondary traumatic stress and burnout, we have been able to distill two primary principles of treatment and prevention that lead to a rapid resolution of symptoms and sustained resilience from future symptoms. These two important principles, which have become the underlying goals for our work in the area of compassion fatigue, are: (1) the development and maintenance of intentionality, through a non-anxious presence, in both personal and professional spheres of life, and (2) the development and maintenance of self-validation, especially self-validated caregiving. We have found, in our own practices and with the caregivers that we have treated, that when these principles are followed not only do negative symptoms diminish, but also quality of life is significantly enhanced and refreshed as new perspectives and horizons begin to open.

Suggestions for Compassion Fatigue Prevention and Resiliency

If you or someone you know is experiencing compassion fatigue symptoms, the following suggestions may be helpful. Please check with your family physician to assure that there are no physical illnesses associated with these symptoms first.

- Become more informed. Read Figley (1995), Stamm (1995) and/or Pearlman & Saakvitne (1995) to learn more about the phenomena of compassion fatigue, vicarious traumatization, and secondary traumatic stress. One book that is especially helpful is *Transforming the Pain: A Workbook on Vicarious Traumatization* by Saakvitne (1996).

- Join a Traumatic Stress Study Group. A weekly, biweekly or monthly meeting of trauma practitioners can become an excellent sanctuary in which the caregiver can both share (therefore diluting) traumatic stories as well as receive support. Check with the ISTSS (*www.istss.org*) for a group that may meet in your area or start one of your own. There are several online support resources also. You can find some of these resources through the excellent David Baldwin's Trauma Pages (*http://www.trauma-pages.com*) in the "Resources" section.

- Begin an exercise program today (see your physician first). Exercise is one of the most important ingredients to effectively manage stress and anxiety and keeps us buoyant and energized while working with heinous trauma.

- Teach your friends and peers how to support you. Don't rely upon random remarks from friends and colleagues to be helpful. Instead, let them know what is most helpful for you during times of stress and pain. You may choose to offer the same to them in a reciprocally supportive arrangement. Periodic or regular professional supervision may also be helpful, especially during a rough time.

- Develop your spirituality. This is different than going to church, although church may be part of your spirituality. Spirituality is your ability to find comfort, support, and meaning from a power greater than yourself. We have found this quality necessary for the development of self-soothing capacity. Meditation, Tai Chi, church/synagogue, Native American rituals, journaling, and workshops are all examples of possible ways in which to enhance one's spirituality.

- Bring your life into balance. Remember that your best is *ALWAYS* good enough. You can only do what you can do so when you leave the office (after 8 hours of work) ... *leave* the office! Perseverating on clients and their situations is not helpful to them, you, or your family. You can help your clients best by refueling and refilling yourself while not at the office. Live your life fully!
- Develop an artistic or sporting discipline. Take lessons and practice as well as play and create. These are integrative and filling experiences. It is paradoxical that when we feel drained that we need to take action instead of sinking into the sedentary „couch potato." Taking action will be rewarded with a greater sense of refreshment and renewal, while activity avoidance will leave us even more vulnerable to the effect of stress the next day.

- Be kind to yourself. If you work with traumatized individuals, families, and/or communities, your life is hard enough already. You do not need to make it more difficult by coercive and critical self-talk. In order to become and remain an effective traumatologist your first responsibility is keeping your instrument in top working condition. Your instrument is *YOU*, and it needs to be cared for.

- Seek short-term treatment. A brief treatment with some of the accelerated trauma techniques (i.e., EMDR) can rapidly resolve secondary traumatic stress symptoms. If you would like assistance in finding a Certified Compassion Fatigue Specialist in your area, please contact the Traumatology Institute at www.psychink.com.

Conclusion

There is little doubt that the extensive efforts being devoted to assisting those affected by the events of September 11, 2001 will have far-reaching influence on the healing of survivors in New York, the people of our nation, and the people of the world. For the first time in the history of our planet, we are beginning to accumulate sufficient knowledge, skills, and resources to facilitate recovery and healing from events such as these. This is not to say that we will not all have painful losses to accommodate or indelible psychological scars – but we will recover. It is a humbling experience to participate, on any level, in this healing.

From our experience with the emergency service workers and professional caregivers who served the survivors of the Murrah building bombing on Oklahoma City since 1995, we also know that there will be casualties in this effort. Many kind and good-hearted emergency service professionals, caregivers, friends, and family members who have witnessed the pain, grief, and terror in their service to survivors will themselves end up wrestling with encroaching intrusive images, thoughts, and feelings from these interactions in the weeks, months, and years ahead.

Compassion fatigue is an area of study that is in its infancy. Therefore, very little empirical research has yet been published in this important area. However, the empirical research that does exist and the stories of hundreds of suffering caregivers provides us with evidence that compassion fatigue, and its painful symptoms, are a very real phenomenon (Deutsch, 1984; McCann & Pearlman, 1990; Follette et al., 1994; Schauben & Frazier, 1995; Cerney, 1995; Salston, 2000). These symptoms carry with them the potential to disrupt, dissolve, and destroy careers, families, and even lives (many of us grieve the loss of at least one colleague who has committed suicide) and should be treated with great respect. Often, it seems, those who suffer most from compassion fatigue are those individuals who are highly motivated to bring about change and healing in the lives of the suffering. It is especially painful to witness the progressive debilitation of these loving caregivers, who are often our very close friends. Without a doubt, many hundreds, if not thousands, of caregivers and emergency service workers providing hour after hour of intensive and life-altering service to those affected by the events of September 11 will experience deleterious effects themselves from this heroic work. Finding the ways and means to both thoroughly study these effects and, maybe more importantly, provide rapidly effective and empirically validated treatment for these suffering heroes, will become a crucial task toward the completion of our nation's healing.

The good news is that the symptoms of compassion fatigue appear to be very responsive to being treated and rapidly ameliorated (Pearlman & Saakvitne, 1995; Gentry & Baranowsky, 1998). While substantially more research in this area will be required before we can offer definitive statements about the nature of treatment, prevention and resiliency with compassion fatigue, some principles and techniques discussed here offer a foundation for helping caregivers resolve their current symptoms and prevent future occurrences. Moreover, we have witnessed that for numerous caregivers the symptoms of compassion fatigue becoming a powerful catalyst for change. With skilled intervention and determination, care providers with compassion fatigue can undergo a profound transformation leaving them more empowered and resilient than they were previously, and therefore better equipped to act as "givers of light."

For more information on compassion fatigue specialist training or treatment, see Appendix 4 of this book.

USING THE TOOLS
Individualized Compassion Fatigue Resiliency Plan

1. **Self Regulation.** Ability to switch from the SNS to the PNS after you have determined that you are safe from threat. Requires relaxation of pelvic (psoas) muscles. Identify two methods that you can employ to relax and keep relaxed this area of your body.

    a. _____

    b. _____

2. **Intentionality.** The ability to follow your mission or "Code of Honor" to within your integrity. The ability to follow the path in which you aim yourself. Identify two areas where you perceive threat, habitually respond reactively, are derailed from your mission, and breech your integrity (can be professional or personal). Make commitment to self-regulate during these periods.

    a. _____

    b. _____

3. **Self-Validated Caregiving.** The ability to give yourself acknowledgement and validation for the work that you do. Resolving the threat perceived and remaining relaxed when client and/or peer is angry or judgmental with you. Ability to monitor and provide self with physical, emotional, and spiritual needs. Identify two situations in your personal or professional life in which you find yourself "caving in" to the perceived demands of a client or peer. Identify situations where you become anxious about the way that you might be perceived by another. Practice relaxation and positive self-supervision in these situations.

    a. _____

    b. _____

4. **Connection/Support.** The employment of three or more peers to serve as a support for you. These persons should be educated in how to best help you and should be able to listen without judgment or interruption. You will want these peers to be "safe" for you and trusted enough that you can share uncomfortable information. These support persons should be used with intention for you to both narrate traumatic experiences (primary and secondary) and expose secrets. Identify three people who you will request to become members of your support family.

    a. _____

    b. _____

    c. _____

Note: These two pages may be reproduced by the purchaser for clinical use.

From: Anna B. Baranowsky, J. Eric Gentry, & D. Franklin Schultz, *Trauma Practice: Tools for Stabilization and Recovery.* © 2011 Hogrefe Publishing

5. **Self-Care.** What activities "refuel" you? You should identify at least one aerobic activity in which you will engage three times weekly. You should also identify an "integrative activity" (e.g., learning a musical instrument, learning an art or craft, learning a sport) that contains both the learning and discipline of mastering the rudiments (e.g., scales, tools, drills) as well as ample time to participate in "playing" in this activity. The remaining three should be activities that replenish you and give you a sense of joy, reconnecting you with life, hope, and wonder. Identify five activities that will help you face each new day with fullness and potency.

a. (aerobic) _____

b. (integrative) _____

c. _____

d. _____

e. _____

That which is to give light

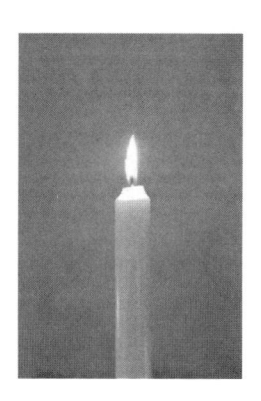

must endure burning

Note: These two pages may be reproduced by the purchaser for clinical use.

From: Anna B. Baranowsky, J. Eric Gentry, & D. Franklin Schultz, *Trauma Practice: Tools for Stabilization and Recovery.* © 2011 Hogrefe Publishing

References

American Psychiatric Association. (2000). *Diagnostic and statistical manual of mental disorders* (4th ed., text revision). Washington, DC: American Psychiatric Association.

Baer, L. (2001). *The imp of the mind.* New York: Dutton.

Baldwin, D. (2004). *David Baldwin's trauma information pages.* [Online resource]. Retrieved from http://www.trauma-pages.com.

Bandler, R., & Grindler, J. (1979). *Frogs into princes.* Moab, UT: Real People Press.

Baranowsky, A. B. (1997). *Layering: A mastery approach to disturbing physical and emotional sensations.* Unpublished manuscript, Toronto: Psych Ink Resources.

Baranowsky, A. B., & Gentry, J. E. (1998a). *Compassion satisfaction manual.* Toronto: Psych Ink Resources.

Baranowsky, A. B., & Gentry, J. E. (1998b). *Workbook/journal for a compassion fatigue specialist.* Toronto: Psych Ink Resources.

Beck, A. T. (1967). *Depression: Causes and treatment.* Philadelphia, PA: University of Pennsylvania Press.

Beck, A. T. (1976). *Cognitive therapy and the emotional disorders.* New York: International Universities Press.

Benson, H. (1997). *The relaxation response.* New York: Avon.

Bercelli, D. (2007). *A bodily approach to trauma recovery.* Retrieved from http://www.traumaprevention.com/index.php?nid=article&article_id=67.

Bercelli, D. (2009). *The revolutionary trauma release process: Transcend your toughest times.* Vancouver: Namaste.

Bergin, A. E., & Garfield, S. L. (1994). The effectiveness of psychotherapy. In A. E. Garfield & S. L. Bergin (Eds.), *Handbook of psychotherapy and behavior change* (pp. 143–189). New York: Wiley.

Bloom, S. L. (2000). Our hearts and our hopes are turned to peace: Origins of the International Society for Traumatic Stress Studies. In A. H. Shalev, R. Yehuda, & A. C. McFarlane (Eds.), *International handbook of human response to trauma* (pp. 27–50). New York: Kluwer Academic/Plenum.

Bonner, R., & Rich, A. (1988). Negative life stress, social problem-solving self-appraisal, and hopelessness: Implications for suicide research. *Cognitive Therapy and Research*, *12*, 549–556.

Bremner, J. D. (2000). The neurobiology of Posttraumatic Stress Disorder. In E. Fink (Ed.), *The encyclopedia of stress* (pp. 186–191). San Diego, CA: Academic Press.

Breslau, N., & Kessler, R. (2001). The stressor criterion in DSM-IV posttraumatic stress disorder: An empirical investigation. *Biological Psychiatry*, *50*, 699–704.

Burns, D. (1980). *Feeling good: The new mood therapy.* New York: Morrow.

Catherall, D. (1995). Coping with secondary traumatic stress: The importance of the therapist's professional peer group. In B. Stamm (Ed.), *Secondary traumatic stress: Self-care issues for clinicians, researchers, and educators* (pp. 80–92). Lutherville, MD: Sidran Press.

Carlson, N. R. (2007). *Physiology of behavior* (9th ed.). Upper Saddle River, NJ: Pearson Education.

Cerney, M. S. (1995). Treating the "heroic treaters". In C. R. Figley (Ed.), *Compassion fatigue: Coping with secondary traumatic stress disorder in those who treat the traumatized* (pp. 131–148). New York: Brunner/Mazel.

Cherniss, C. (1980). *Professional burnout in human service organizations.* New York: Praeger.

Cloitre, M. (1998). Sexual revictimization: Risk factors and prevention. In V. M. Follette, J. I. Ruzek, & F. R. Abeug (Eds.), *Cognitive-behavioral therapies for trauma* (pp. 278–304). New York: Guilford.

Committee on Treatment of Posttraumatic Stress Disorder, National Institute of Medicine. (2008). *Treatment of posttraumatic stress disorder: An assessment of the evidence.* Washington, DC: National Academies Press.

Covey, S. R., Merrill, A. R., & Merrill, R. R. (1977). *First things first.* New York: Simon & Schuster.

Cox, C. L. (1992). Perceived threat as a cognitive component of state anxiety and confidence. *Perception and Motor Skills*, *75*, 1092–1094.

Critchley, H. C., Melmed, R. N., Featherstone, E., Mathias, C. J., & Dolan, R. J. (2001). Brain activity during biofeedback relaxation. *Brain: A Journal of Neurology*, *124*, 1003–1012.

Danieli, Y. (1982). Psychotherapists participation in the conspiracy of silence about the Holocaust. *Psychoanalytic Psychology*, *1*, 23–46.

Deutsch, C. J. (1984). Self-reported sources of stress among psychotherapists. *Professional Psychology: Research & Practice*, *15*, 833–845.

Dolan, Y. M. (1991). *Resolving sexual abuse: Solution-focused therapy and ericksonian hypnosis for adult survivors.* New York: Norton.

Doublet, S. (2000). *The stress myth.* Chesterfield, MO: Science & Humanities Press.

Ehrenreich, J. H. (1999). *Coping with disaster: A guidebook to psychosocial intervention* [Online]. Retrieved from http://www.mhwwb.org/contents.htm.

Ellis, A., & Harper, R. A. (1961). *A guide to rational living.* Englewood Cliffs, NJ: Prentice-Hall.

Erickson, M. H., & Rossi, E. L. (1989). *The February man.* New York: Brunner/Mazel.

Falconer, E. M. (2008). *Inhibitory control in posttraumatic stress disorder (PTSD).* Defended dissertation at University of New South Wales. http://handle.unsw.edu.au/1959.4/40156.

Farber, B. A. (1983). Introduction: A critical perspective on burnout. In B. A. Farber (Ed.), *Stress and burnout in the human service professions* (pp. 1–20). New York: Pergamon.

Figley, C. R. (1983). Catastrophe: An overview of family reactions. In C. R. Figley & H. I. McCubbin (Eds.), *Stress and the family: Vol. II. Coping with catastrophe.* New York: Brunner/Mazel.

Figley, C. R. (1988). Toward a field of traumatic stress. *Journal of Traumatic Stress, 1,* 3–16.

Figley, C. R. (1995). *Compassion fatigue: Coping with secondary traumatic stress disorder in those who treat the traumatized.* New York: Brunner/Mazel.

Figley, C. R. (Ed.). (2002) *Treating compassion fatigue.* New York: Brunner-Routledge.

Figley, C., Bride, B. E., & Mazza, N. (Eds.). (1997). *Death and trauma: The traumatology of grieving.* Washington: Taylor & Francis.

Figley, C. R., & Kleber, R. (1995). Beyond the "victim": Secondary traumatic stress. In R. J. Kleber & C. R. Figley (Eds.), *Beyond trauma: Cultural and societal dynamics* (pp. 75–98). New York: Plenum.

Figley, C. R., & Stamm, B. H. (1996). Psychometric review of Compassion Fatigue Self Test. In B. H. Stamm (Ed.), *Measurement of stress, trauma and adaptation* (pp. 127–130). Lutherville, MD: Sidran Press.

Foa, E. B., Dancu, C. V., Hembree, E. A., Jaycox, L. A., Meadows, E. A., & Street, G. P. (1999). The efficacy of exposure therapy, stress inoculation training and their combination in ameliorating PTSD for female victims of assault. *Journal of Consulting and Clinical Psychology, 67,* 194–200.

Foa, E. B., Davidson, J. R. T., & Frances, A. (1999). The Expert Consensus Guideline Series: Treatment of Posttraumatic Stress Disorder. *The Journal of Clinical Psychiatry, 60,* Suppl. 16.

Foa, E. B., Keane, T. M., & Friedman, M. J. (Eds.). (2000). *Effective treatments for PTSD.* New York: Guilford.

Foa, E. B., & Meadows, E. A. (1997). Psychosocial treatments for posttraumatic stress disorder: A critical review. *Annual Review of Psychology, 48,* 449–480.

Follette, V. M., Polusny, M. M., & Milbeck, K. (1994). Mental health and law enforcement professionals: Trauma history, psychological symptoms, and impact of providing services to sexual abuse survivors. *Professional Psychology: Research and Practice, 25,* 275–282.

Follette, V. M., Ruzek, J. I., & Abueg, F. R. (1998). *Cognitive behavioral therapies for trauma.* New York: Guilford.

Frankl, V. E. (1963). *Man's search for meaning.* New York: Washington Square Press, Simon and Schuster.

French, G. D., & Harris, C. (1998). *Traumatic incident reduction (TIR).* Boca Raton, FL: CRC Press.

Freudenberger, H. (1974). Staff burn-out. *Journal of Social Issues, 30,* 159–165.

Friedman, M. J. (1996). PTSD diagnosis and treatment for mental health clinicians. *Community Mental Health Journal, 32,* 173–189.

Gentry, J. E. (1999). The trauma recovery scale (TRS): An outcome measure. Poster session presented at the meeting of the International Society for Traumatic Stress Studies, Miami, FL.

Gentry, J. E. (2000). *Certified compassion fatigue specialist training: Training-as-treatment.* Unpublished dissertation, Florida State University.

Gentry, J. E. (2002). Compassion fatigue: A crucible of transformation. *The Journal of Trauma Practice, 1,* 37–61.

Gentry, J. E., & Baranowsky, A. B. (1998). *Treatment manual for the Accelerated Recovery Program: Set II.* Toronto: Psych Ink Resources.

Gentry, J. E., & Baranowsky, A. B. (1999a). *Compassion satisfaction manual: 1-Day group workshop, Set III-B.* Toronto: Psych Ink Resources.

Gentry, J. E., & Baranowsky, A. B. (1999b). *Compassion satisfaction manual: 2-Day group retreat, Set III-C.* Toronto: Psych Ink Resources.

Gentry, J. E., & Baranowsky, A. B. (1999, November). *Accelerated Recovery Program for Compassion Fatigue.* Preconference workshop presented at the 15th Annual meeting of the International Society for Traumatic Stress Studies, Miami, FL.

Gentry, J. E., Baranowsky, A. B., & Dunning, K. (2002). The Accelerated Recovery Program (ARP) for Compassion Fatigue. In C. R. Figley (Ed.), *Treating compassion fatigue.* New York: Brunner-Routledge.

George, M. S., Sackeim, H. A., Rush, A. J., Marangell, L. B., Nahas, Z., Husain, M. M., Lisanby, S., Burt, T., Goldman, J., & Ballenger, J. C. (2000). Vagus nerve stimulation: a new tool for brain research and therapy. *Biological Psychiatry, 47,* 287–295.

Gold, S. N., & Faust, J. (2001). The future of trauma practice: Visions and aspirations. *Journal of Trauma Practice, 1,* 1–15.

Goldberg, E. (2001). *The executive brain: Frontal lobes and the civilized mind.* New York: Oxford Press.

Grinder, J., & Bandler, R. (1981). *Trance-formations: Neuro-linquistic programming and the structure of hypnosis.* Moab, UT: Real People Press.

Grosch, W. N., & Olsen, D. C. (1994). Therapist burnout: A self psychology and systems perspective. In W. N. Grosch & D. C. Olsen (Eds.), *When helping starts to hurt: A new look at burnout among psychotherapists* (pp. 439–454). New York: Norton.

Haley, S. (1974). When the patient reports atrocities. *Archives of General Psychiatry, 39,* 191–196.

Hamarat, E., Thompson, D., Zabrucky, K. M., Steele, D., Matheny, K. B., & Aysan, F. (2001). Perceived stress and coping resource availability as predictors of life satisfaction in young, middle-aged, and older adults. *Experimental Aging Research, 27,* 181–196.

Hanh, T. N. (1990). *The path of mindfulness in everyday life.* New York: Bantam.

Heim, C., Ehlert, U., Hanker, J. P., & Hellhammer, D. H. (1998). Abuse-related posttraumatic stress disorder and alterations of the hypothalamic-pituitary-adrenal axis in women with chronic pelvic pain. *Psychosomatic Medicine, 60,* 309–331.

Herman, J. L. (1981). *Father-daughter incest.* Cambridge, MA: Harvard University Press.

Herman, J. L. (1992). *Trauma and recovery.* New York: Basic Books.

Holbrook, T. L., Hoyt, D. B., Stein, M. B., & Sieber, W. J. (2001). Perceived threat to life predicts posttraumatic stress disorder after major trauma: risk factors and functional outcome. *The Journal of Trauma: Injury, Infection, and Critical Care, 51,* 287–293.

Holland, J. C., Morrow, G. R., Schmale, J., Derogatis, L., Stefanek, M., Berenson, S., Carpenter, P. J., Breitbart, W., & Feldstein, M. (1991). A randomized clinical trial of alprazolam versus progressive muscle relaxation in cancer patients with anxiety and depressive symptoms. *Journal of Clinical Oncology, 9,* 1004–1011.

Holmes, D., & Tinnin, L. (1995). The problem of auditory hallucinations in combat PTSD. *Traumatology - e: On-line Electronic Journal of Trauma, 1.* Retrieved from http://www.fsu.edu/~trauma/art1v1i2.html.

International Society for Traumatic Stress Studies, ISTSS. (n.d.). Resources for the public. Retrieved from http://www.istss.org/resources/index.cfm.

Jamison, R. N. (1996). *Mastering chronic pain: A professional's guide to behavioral treatment.* New York: Professional Resource Exchange.

Johnson, S. (2003, March 1). Emotions and the brain: Fear. *Discover: Science, Technology, and the Future.* Retrieved March 5, 2009, from http://www.discovermagazine.com/2003/mar/cover.

Jung, C. G. (1907). The pychology of dementia praecox. In H. Read, M. Fordham, G. Adler, & W. McGuire (Eds.), *The collected works of C. G. Jung, Vol. 3* (Bollingen Series XX). Princeton, NJ: Princeton University Press.

Kabat-Zinn, J. (1990). *Full catastrophe living: Using the wisdom of your body and mind to face stress, pain, and illness.* New York: Delta.

Karakashian, M. (1994). Countertransference issues in crisis work with natural disaster victims. *Psychotherapy, 31,* 334–341.

Kegel, A. H. (1951). Physiologic therapy for urinary stress incontinence. *Journal of the American Medical Association, 146,* 915–917.

Kinsella, S. M., & Tuckey, J. P. (2001). Perioperative bradycardia and asystole: relationship to vasovagal syncope and the Bezold – Jarisch reflex. *British Journal of Anaesthesia, 86,* 859–868.

Krost, B. (2007). Understanding and releasing the psoas muscle. Retrieved from http://www.naturalreflexes.com/pages/psoas.html.

Lim, S. H., Anantharaman, V., Goh, P. P., & Tan, A. T. (1998). Comparrison of treatment of supraventricular tachycardia by Valsalva maneuver and carotid sinus massage. *Annals of Emergency Medicine, 31,* 30–35.

Lindy, J. D. (1988). *Vietnam: A casebook.* New York: Brunner/Mazel.

Luecken, L., Dausch, B., Gulla, V., Hong, R., Compas, B. (2004). Alterations in morning cortisol associated with PTSD in women with breast cancer. Journal of Psychosomatic Research, 56, 13–15.

Mandle, C. L., Jacobs, S. C., Acari, P. M., Domar, A. D. (1998). The efficacy of relaxation response interventions with adult patients: A review of the literature. In C. E. Guzzetta (Ed.), *Essential readings in holistic nursing* (pp. 243–263). New York: Aspen.

Mason, J. W., Giller, E. L., Kosten, T. R., Harkness, L. (1988). Elevation of urinary norepinephrine/cortisol ratio in posttraumatic stress disorder. *Journal of Nervous and Mental Disease, 176,* 498–502.

Marmar, C. R., Weiss, D. S., Metzler, T. J., Delucchi, K. L., Best, S. R., & Wentworth, K. A. (1999). Longitudinal course and predictors of continuing distress following critical incident exposure in emergency services personnel. *Journal of Nervous and Mental Disease, 187,* 15–22.

Maslach, C. (1976). Burnout. *Human Behavior, 5,* 16–22.

Maslach, C. (1982). Understanding burnout: Definitional issues in analyzing a complex phenomenon. In W. S. Paine (Ed.), *Job stress and burnout: Research, theory and intervention perspectives* (pp. 29–30). Beverly Hills, CA: Sage.

Maslach, C., & Goldberg, J. (1998). Prevention of burnout: New perspectives. *Applied and Preventive Psychology, 7,* 63–74.

Matsakis, A. (1994). *Vietnam wives: Facing the challenges of life with veterans suffering post-traumatic stress.* New York: Basic Books.

McCann, I. L., & Pearlman, L. A. (1990). Vicarious traumatization: A framework for understanding the psychological effects of working with victims. *Journal of Traumatic Stress, 3,* 131–149.

McNally, V. (1998). Training of FBI employee assistance professionals and chaplains at FBI Headquarters. Washington, DC, November 7–8.

McNaughton, N. (1997). Cognitive dysfunction resulting from hippocampal hyperactivity – A possible cause of anxiety disorder? *Pharmacology Biochemistry and Behavior, 56,* 603–611.

Meichenbaum, D. (1994). *A clinical handbook/practical therapist manual: For assessing and treating adults with Post-Traumatic Stress Disorder (PTSD).* Waterloo, Canada: University of Waterloo – Institute Press.

Mitchell, J. (1995). The critical incident stress debriefing (CISD) and the prevention of work-related traumatic stress among high risk occupational groups. In G. Everly (Ed.), *Psycho-traumatology: Key papers and core concepts in post-traumatic stress* (pp. 267–280). New York: Plenum.

Mower, O. H. (1960). *Learning theory and behavior.* New York: Wiley.

Norman, J. (2001). The brain, the bucket, and the schwoop. In J. E. Gentry (Ed.) *Traumatology 1001: Field traumatology training manual* (pp. 34–37). Tampa, FL: International Traumatology Institute.

Pearlman, L. A. (1995). Self-care for trauma therapists: Ameliorating vicarious traumatization. In B. H. Stamm (Ed.), *Secondary traumatic stress: Self-care issues for clinicians, researchers, and educators* (pp. 51–64). Lutherville, MD: Sidran.

Pearlman, L. A., & Saakvitne, K. W. (1995). *Trauma and the therapist: Countertransference and vicarious traumatization in psychotherapy with incest survivors.* New York: Norton.

Perry, B. D. (2007). Self-regulation: The second core strength. Retrieved from http://teacher.scholastic.com/professional/bruceperry/self_regulation.htm#bio.

Pole, N., Best, S. R., Weiss, D. S., Metzler, T. J., Liberman, A. M., Fagan, J., & Marmar, C. R. (2001). Effects of gender and ethnicity on duty-related posttraumatic stress symptoms among urban police officers. *Journal of Nervous and Mental Disease, 189,* 442–448.

Porges, S. (1992). Vagal tone: A physiologic marker of stress vulnerability. *Pediatrics, 90,* 498–504.

Porges, S. (1999). Emotions: An evolutionary by-product of the neural regulation of the autonomic nervous system. In C. S. Carter, I. I. Lederhendler, and B. Kirpatrick (Eds.), *The integrative biology of affiliation.* Cambridge, MA: MIT Press.

Resick, P. A., & Schnicke, M. K. (1992). Cognitive processing therapy for sexual assault victims. *Journal of Consulting and Clinical Psychology, 60,* 748–756.

Resick, P. A., & Schnicke, M. K. (1993). *Cognitive processing therapy for rape victims: A treatment manual.* Newbury Park, CA: Sage.

Rothbaum, B. O., Meadows, E. A., Resick, P., & Foy, D. W. (2000). Cognitive-Behavioral Therapy. In E. B. Foa, T. M. Keane, & M. J. Friedman (Eds.), *Effective treatments for PTSD* (pp. 60–83). New York: Guilford.

Rothschild, B. (2000). *The body remembers: The psychophysiology of trauma and trauma treatment.* New York: Norton.

Saakvitne, K. W., & Pearlman, L. A. (Eds.) (1996). *Transforming the pain: A workbook on vicarious traumatization.* New York: Norton.

Salston, M. D. (1999). *Compassion fatigue: Implications for mental health professionals and trainees.* A defended critical review at Florida State University.

Salston, M. D. (2000). *Secondary traumatic stress: A study exploring empathy and the exposure to the traumatic material of survivors of community violence.* Defended dissertation, Florida State University.

Sapolsky, R. M., (2004). *Why zebras don't get ulcers* (3rd ed.). New York: Holt.

Scaer, R. C. (2001). *The body bears the burden: Trauma, dissociation, and disease.* Binghamton, NY: Hawthorne.

Scaer, R.C. (2006). *The trauma spectrum: Hidden wounds, human resiliency.* New York: Basic Books.

Schauben, L. J., & Frazier, P. A., (1995). Vicarious trauma: The effects on female counselors of working with sexual violence survivors. *Psychology of Women Quarterly, 19,* 49–64.

Schnarch, D. M. (1991). *Constructing the sexual crucible: An integration of sexual and marital therapy.* New York: Norton.

Schultz, D. F. (2004). *A language of the heart: Therapy stories that heal.* Highland City, FL: Rainbow Books.

Schultz, D. F. (2005). *A language of the heart workbook.* Highland City, FL: Rainbow Books

Schnurr, P. P., Lunney, C. A., Sengupta, A. (2004). Risk factors for the development versus maintenance of posttraumatic stress disorder. *Journal of Trauma Stress, 17,* 85–95.

References

Sedgewick, D. (1995). Countertransference from a Jungian perspective (transcript of a lecture given at Grand Rounds to the Department of Psychiatric Medicine, University of Virginia). The C. G. Jung Page, http://www.cgjung.com/articles/roundsx.html.

Sexton, L. (1999). Vicarious traumatization of counselors and effects on their workplaces. *British Journal of Guidance and Counseling, 27,* 393–403.

Shalev, A., Bonne, O., & Eth, S. (1996). Treatment of posttraumatic stress disorder: A review. *Psychosomatic Medicine, 58,* 165–182.

Shapiro, F. (1989). Efficacy of the eye movement desensitization procedure: A new treatment for posttraumatic stress disorder. *Journal of Traumatic Stress, 2,* 199–223.

Shapiro, F. (1995). *Eye movement desensitization and reprocessing: Basic principles, protocols and procedures.* New York: Guilford.

Shusterman, V., & Barnea, O. (2005). Sympathetic nervous system activity in stress and biofeedback relaxation. *Engineering in Medicine and Biology Magazine, IEEE, 24,* 52–57.

Sikirov, B. A. (1990). Cardio-vascular events at defecation: are they unavoidable? *Medical Hypothesis, 32,* 231–233.

Spilsbury, J. C., Belliston, L., Drotar, D., Drinkard, A., Kretschmar, J., Creeden, R., Flannery, D. J., & Friedman, S. (2006). Clinically significant trauma symptoms and behavioral problems in a community-based sample of children exposed to domestic violence. *Journal of Family Violence, 22,* 487–499.

Stamm, B. H. (1995). *Secondary traumatic stress: Self-care issues for clinicians, researchers, and educators.* Lutherville, MD: Sidran Press.

Stoppelbein, L. A., Greening, L., & Elkin, T. D. (2006). Risk of posttraumatic stress symptoms: A comparison of child survivors of pediatric cancer and parental bereavement. *Journal of Pediatric Psychology, 31,* 367–376.

Sussman, M. (1992). *A curious calling: Unconscious motivations for practicing psychotherapy.* Northvale, NJ: Aronson.

Takahashi, T., Ikeda, K., Ishikawa, M., Kitamura, N., Tsukasaki, T., Nakama, D. & Kameda, T. (2005). Anxiety, reactivity, and social stress-induced cortisol elevation in humans. *Neuroendocrinology Letters, 4,* 351–354.

Tinnin, L. (1994). *Time-limited trauma therapy: A treatment manual.* Bruceton Mills, WV: Gargoyle.

van der Kolk, B. (1996). The black hole of trauma. In B. A. van der Kolk, A. C. McFarlane, & L. Weisaeth (Eds.). *Traumatic stress: The effects of overwhelming experience on mind, body, and society* (pp. 3–23). New York: Guilford.

van der Kolk, B. A., McFarlane, A. C., & Weisaeth, L. (Eds.). (1996). *Traumatic stress: The effects of overwhelming experience on mind, body, and society.* New York: Guilford.

Waxman, M. B., Wald, R. W., Finley, J. P., Bonet, J. F., Downar, E.. & Sharma, A. D. (1980). Valsalva termination of ventricular tachycardia. *Circulation, 62,* 843–851.

Wilson, J., & Lindy, J. (1994). *Countertransference in the treatment of PTSD.* New York: Guilford.

Wolpe, J. (1958). *Psychotherapy by reciprocal inhibition.* Stanford, CA: Stanford University Press.

Wolpe, J. (1969). *The practice of behavioral therapy.* New York: Pergamon.

World Health Organization. (2007). *The world health report 2007 – A safer future: global public health security in the 21st century*. Retrieved from http://www.who.int/whr/2007/en/index.html.

Yartz, A. R., & Hawk, L. W. (2001) Psychophysiological assessment of anxiety: Tales from the heart. In M. Antony, S. Orsillo, & L. Roemer (Eds.), Practitioner's guide to empirically based measures of anxiety (pp. 25–30). New York: Springer.

Yehuda, R. (2001). Biology of posttraumatic stress disorder. *Journal of Clinical Psychiatry, 62,* 41–46.

Appendices

Appendix 1
Self-Regulation

Transformation: From Sympathetic to Parasympathetic

Recent brain imaging research has begun to demonstrate that anxiety is a brain killer – the more anxiety a person experiences, the less effectively our brains operate. It is becoming increasing apparent that professional and personal effectiveness require self-regulation skills. By relaxing the muscles of the pelvic region (i.e., kegels, sphincter, and psoas), we are able to affect profound systemic muscle relaxation. This relaxation facilitates a shift in the autonomous nervous system (ANS) from the *sympathetic* system (i.e., fight-or-flight reflex utilized during periods of perceived threat) to the *parasympathetic* system (i.e., relaxation and optimal functioning utilized during period of safety). By maintaining this pelvic relaxation, we are able to thwart the ANS from shifting to sympathetic dominance each time we perceive even the mildest threats (e.g., criticism).

By practicing the release and relaxation of these muscles, we can gradually shift from sympathetic to parasympathetic dominance. The rewards of this transformation include comfort in our bodies, maximal motor and cognitive functioning, ability to tolerate intimacy, self-regulation, internal vs. external locus of control, ability to remain mission/principle driven, increased tolerance, increased effectiveness, and increased health of our body's systems.

What happens when my sympathetic nervous system is dominant?

When you perceive a threat, your body responds to either neutralize or move away from this perceived threat. This is true for all species of living things and is known as the fight-or-flight reflex. If we are truly in danger of losing our lives, then this reflex is arguably useful. However, we are rarely confronted with threats and circumstances that are this dire in our daily lives. Instead, we perceive some mild threat, our sympathetic nervous system (SNS) activates, and we find ourselves trying to either kill or run away from our boss, coworker, or spouse. This overactive and very sensitive threat identification and early warning system is the cause of all stress.

When our SNS is activated and dominant, we are preparing for battle or flight. Our circulation becomes constricted, our heart rate increases, and our muscles become tense and ready to act. Inside our brains, the neocortex becomes less functional while the brain stem, basal ganglia, and thalamus become more active. This is because the perceived need to survive has superseded all other brain functioning. As we become more stressed, and the longer we are in this state of sympathetic dominance, the more likely we are to compromise the functioning of higher-order brain systems such as language, speech, motor activity, filtering, and compassion. This loss of functioning may partially account for why people have trouble thinking logically during stressful times, or why they have trouble being kind when they perceive threat, or even why they have trouble with peak physical performance (e.g., sports) when they are "nervous." By simply relaxing and keeping relaxed our pelvic muscles we can reverse this process of sympathetic dominance and return to parasympathetic systems. This return to parasympathetic dominance will allow the individual to regain optimal functioning of speech, language (remember intentional thought is simply talking to ourselves – something for which we need to be able to create language and speech), motor coordination, filtering, and compassion. Once an individual is able to successfully transition from sympathetic to parasympathetic dominance, without external agents (i.e., drugs) and without regard for the external events (i.e., crises) the individual has become self-regulatory. A person who becomes skilled in making this transition has developed an internal locus of control and is no longer a victim of circumstances.

Where are the pelvic muscles? How do I find them?

While conducting seminars students often ask me this question. I cannot help but feel a twinge of sadness when this question is asked. The sadness comes from the awareness that the person asking this question has learned to be unaware of these muscles. People who are not aware of the muscles in their midbody are not aware for good reason – it has been a coping strategy since childhood. Children who grew up in anxious and dangerous environments learned to keep their bodies tight in anticipation of danger. With no skills for self-regulating, these children often learn to numb and dissociate their awareness away from the pain in their bodies. These children grow into adults that have difficulty being "in" their bodies – they have difficultly monitoring and regulating muscle tension and, ultimately, anxiety.

Exercise

1. While sitting, put your hands under your butt.
2. Feel the two pointed bones upon which you are sitting.
3. Now, touch the two bony points on your right and left side just below the waist.
4. You have made a touch memory for four distinct points. Connect those four points to make a square.
5. Now, allow your breath to get to the area in the middle of the square. Also, allow the square to expand.
6. Release and relax all muscles that traverse the area of the square so that there are *no clenched muscles* in the square.

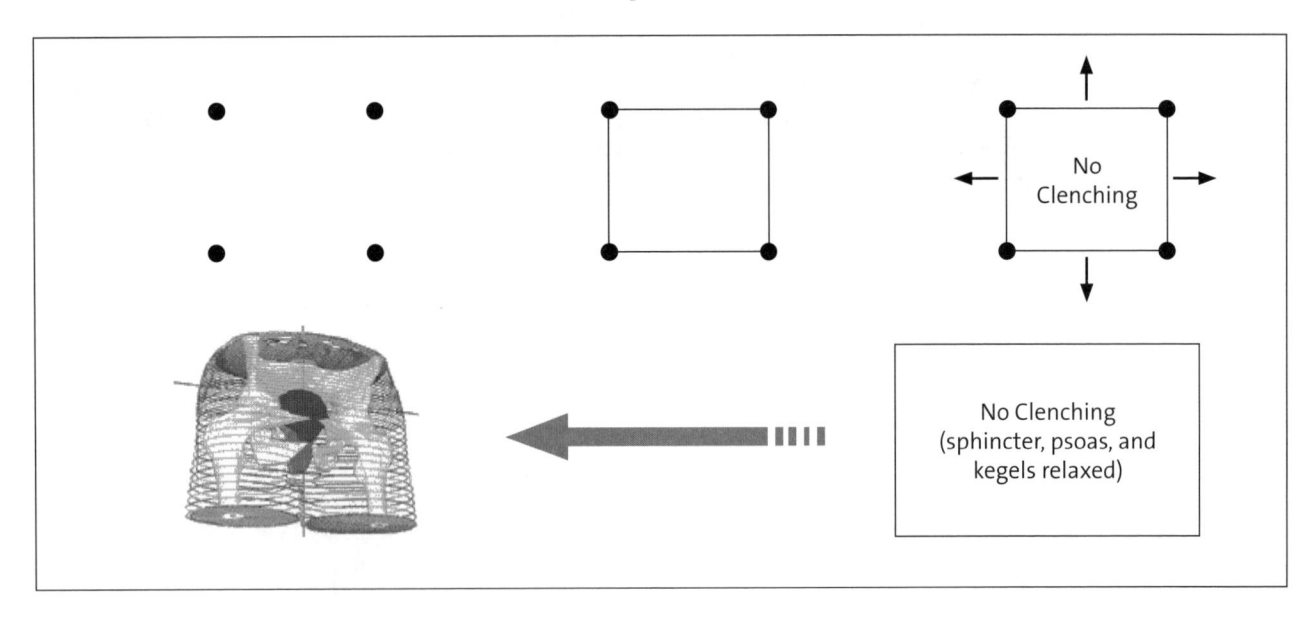

What now that my pelvic muscles are relaxed?

Keep them that way. If you are able to keep your pelvic muscles released and relaxed for 20 – 30 seconds, then you will begin to notice the clear differences in yourself as you transition from sympathetic to parasympathetic dominance. You will first notice comfort in your body. As you release the tension and stress that you have been generating you will become aware that your body is comfortable – no matter what is going on around you. Your thoughts may still be racing and producing warning messages. If this is happening, *do nothing*; just concentrate on keeping your pelvic muscles relaxed. This will be difficult for many people because, since childhood, we have taken action when we experience this alarm. However, if we are able to keep our pelvic muscles relaxed then we will be rewarded with a lessening of stress and the restoration of optimal functioning in our thinking and actions. With this self-regulation, we will be able to comfortably seek creative solutions to problems and situations that used to leave us baffled, exhausted, and frustrated.

By developing and practicing the skills of self-regulation we will find ourselves able to maintain fidelity to our intention – our mission. We will find that we no longer need to react to every little crisis as though it is a life-or-death situation. We will become free from our pasts to live for ourselves the lives that we create without having to be perpetually "on guard" for the next danger. We will be able to function at peak effectiveness anytime we choose – a transformation indeed.

Sympathetic = Reactive = Stress = Diminished Functioning = No Choice
Parasympathetic = Intentional = Comfort = Optimal Functioning = Choice

You Choose

Appendix 2
Pinnacle Exercises

Living a Principle-Based Life: Foundation Exercises

To build a great building, much care must go into both planning and constructing the foundation of that building. The same is true for building a great life. For those who have decided to embark upon developing and maintaining a life that is lived according to principles, instead of the capricious whims of circumstances and the impossibility of unachievable outcomes, then you must first become intimate with your own principles.

Compassion Unlimited has developed three important exercises that will help you make these values and principles explicit so that you can begin to intentionally live in accordance with them. By completing the enclosed Vision Statement, Covenant, and Code of Honor Exercises, you will have developed the important foundation of your principle-based life. The Vision Statement Exercise will help you to clarify where you are going – the outcomes and final destinations of a principle-based life. The Covenant Exercise will take you on a journey through your life up to the present, helping you to extract the important elements, affinities, and expertise to articulate the purpose of your life – your Covenant. Finally, the Code of Honor Exercise will guide you through the selection of 10–12 principles that become the pathway for your mission – the tenets of your integrity – and will help you to accelerate the achievement of your goals.

All future work in the Pinnacle Program will utilize the fruits of these exercises to help you maintain fidelity to your principles. By maintaining this fidelity, you assure yourself that you are traveling the fastest and simplest path toward achieving your vision. The tools and skills you will learn and practice during your work with the program will aid you in overcoming the obstacles that have previously slowed or thwarted you in your attempts to achieve your vision.

Give yourself an hour or so of uninterrupted and relaxed time to complete the next few pages of exercises. You are creating the foundation for your new life, so be intentional with your words. However, you will always be able to change, edit, update each of the three documents you are about to write – knowing that they are organic and will continue to change and evolve. Do your best and it will be a perfect place for us to start our work.

Vision Statement Exercise

Your vision statement is an extremely important tool in developing and maintaining a principle-based life. Your vision describes the outcome and payoff of all your hard work. It is where you will end up if you follow your mission and stay true to your principles. Your vision articulates who you are and what you are doing when you are where you want to be. This exercise is designed to help you articulate your vision.

Preparation

Complete the Mission Statement Exercise before writing your Vision Statement. You will be able to cull many of the principles and language for your Vision Statement from this previous exercise. Use the "Retirement Party Visualization" exercise from the CD *The Accelerated Recovery Program for Compassion Fatigue: A Self-Guided Resiliency & Recovery Series* (Baranowsky & Gentry, 2002. Psych Ink Resources,. http://www.psychink.com). This exercise will help you visualize yourself at your own retirement party and allows you to "see" yourself having already arrived at your vision. This exercise is an excellent way to stimulate your thinking and emotions toward writing a perfect vision statement.

If you are unable to acquire the CD, then take a few moments (10–15 minutes) to clear your mind and begin to imagine yourself getting where you want to be, doing what you want to do, and, most importantly, being the person that you want to be. Jot down a few notes.

Suggestions:
- A vision statement should be contained within a 2–5 sentence paragraph, written in the present tense (e.g., "I am financially secure" instead of "I will achieve financial security").
- A vision statement should be global instead of specific (e.g., "I am a national leader in the field of financial planning" instead of "I have 450 active clients").
- A vision statement should be written in the first person (e.g., "I am a successful and respected corporate attorney").
- A vision statement is your achievable dream – your carrot dangling from a stick that keeps you moving and on track. Make certain that the vision statement you write provides you with sufficient motivation and inspiration to keep you committed to your mission during the lean and difficult times.
- Your vision statement articulates you achieving and fulfilling the purpose of your life – the reason for your being.
- Make certain that your vision statement is for you – not your spouse, your parents, your children, or your boss.
- Write your vision statement without regard to fear or risk (who would you be if you never experienced fear?).
- Remember that the better you know yourself and your mission, the more refined your mission will become. Write your vision today with all the information you have available to you, knowing that it may change tomorrow. There is no "wrong" way to write a vision statement.

Covenant Exercise

A Covenant is designed to provide its author with direction, purpose, and motivation toward actualizing all of their potentials – both professional and personal. It is written in an active and declarative voice and should empower its writer with a clear vision of their "best self" – the person they are becoming. This exercise is designed to help you bring into focus this best self and to identify pathways to facilitate the continued evolution toward this goal.

An empowering Covenant
1. represents the deepest and best within you. It comes out of a solid connection with your deep inner life.
2. is the fulfillment of your own unique gifts. It is the expression of your unique capacity to contribute.
3. is transcendent. It is based on principles of contribution and purpose higher than self.
4. addresses and integrates all four fundamental human needs and capacities. It includes fulfillment in physical, social, mental, and spiritual dimensions.
5. is based on principles that produce quality-of-life results. Both the ends and the means are based on true north principles.
6. deals with both vision and principle-based values. It is not good enough to have values without vision – you want to be good, but you want to be good for something. On the other hand, vision without values can produce a Hitler. An empowering mission statement deals with both character and competence – what you want to be and what you want to do in your life.
7. deals with all significant roles in your life. It represents a lifetime balance of personal, family, work, community – whatever roles are yours to fill.
8. is written to inspire you, not impress anyone else. It communicates to you and inspires you at the most elemental level. (Covey, 1997, p. 107)

USING THE TOOLS
Preparation

Time-limited exercise. Take five minutes and complete the following questions:

a. Why are you alive? What is your purpose for being on this planet?
___
___
___

b. What do you want to be when you grow up?
___
___
___

c. What dreams do you have for yourself that are yet unfulfilled?
___
___
___

d. What do you want to be when you grow up?{AU: Identical to question (b). Please verify.}
___
___
___

e. What are your greatest strengths?
___
___
___

Stop. Review the above answers and circle the top five in each category. What does this tell you about yourself? Where are you in alignment with your values and principles? Where are you out of alignment? Take a moment to simply write down your thoughts after reviewing the above answers:
___
___
___

Note: This page may be reproduced by the purchaser for clinical use.

From: Anna B. Baranowsky, J. Eric Gentry, & D. Franklin Schultz, *Trauma Practice: Tools for Stabilization and Recovery*. © 2011 Hogrefe Publishing

USING THE TOOLS
Practice
(Adapted from Covey, Merrill, & Merrill, 1997)

Practice with the following sentence forms to start creating your vision and mission for yourself. Take one minute to complete each unfinished sentence.

It is my covenant:

To live: _____

_____

_____

To work: _____

_____

_____

To continue: _____

_____

_____

To love: _____

_____

_____

To be: _____

_____

_____

To become: _____

_____

_____

Note: These two pages may be reproduced by the purchaser for clinical use.

From: Anna B. Baranowsky, J. Eric Gentry, & D. Franklin Schultz, *Trauma Practice: Tools for Stabilization and Recovery.* © 2011 Hogrefe Publishing

To believe: _____
_____
_____

To promote: _____
_____
_____

To strive: _____
_____
_____

To seek: _____
_____
_____

Now write your covenant

Note: These two pages may be reproduced by the purchaser for clinical use.

From: Anna B. Baranowsky, J. Eric Gentry, & D. Franklin Schultz, *Trauma Practice: Tools for Stabilization and Recovery.* © 2011 Hogrefe Publishing

USING THE TOOLS
My Covenant

Code of Honor Exercise

This exercise is the last of three in helping you establish the foundations of a principle-based life. If your vision statement represents the destination of your life and your mission statement represents your purpose, then your principles are the methods that you utilize to perform your mission and to achieve your vision. Your principles articulate your integrity – the laws and rules that you will choose to live by. Using a train metaphor, your vision statement is the destination, your mission statement is the train and its fuel, and your principles are the tracks upon which the train glides. The better you are at remaining on the tracks of your principles, avoiding derailment, the more quickly and effortlessly you will achieve your vision.

My Principles

Below is a list of words that can be constructed into "Code of Honor" principle-based statements (example: Honest = "I am honest in all dealings with others and myself").

Honest	Conservative	Effective
Challenging	Liberal	Scientific
Approach vs. avoidance	Moderate	Creative
Ethical	Tolerant	Detailed
Frugal	Conservative	Compassionate
Faithful	Outspoken	Resilient
Sense of humor	Assertive	Powerful
Commitment	Service	Responsible
Hopeful	Greedy	Productive
Joyous	Efficient	Just
Courage	Leader	Passionate
Truth/truthful	Facilitative	Secure
Parenting	Optimistic	Loving
Non-violent/peaceable	Farsighted	Strong
Fearless	Self-confident	Active

Pick 10–12 words from the above list and write sentences that describe you living these principles perfectly all the time (e.g., "I remain hopeful in all situations"). It is understood that you will not be able to maintain these principles 100% of the time and is the focus of our work. You will, however, become progressively more efficient in living within your principles as you practice some of the tools you will learn in the Pinnacle Program. Remember, with this exercise you are laying the tracks toward your vision upon which you will practice your mission day in and day out. – Make certain that the principles you choose are really the right ones for you.

To thine own self be true.

Appendix 3
Reactive to Intentional Worksheet

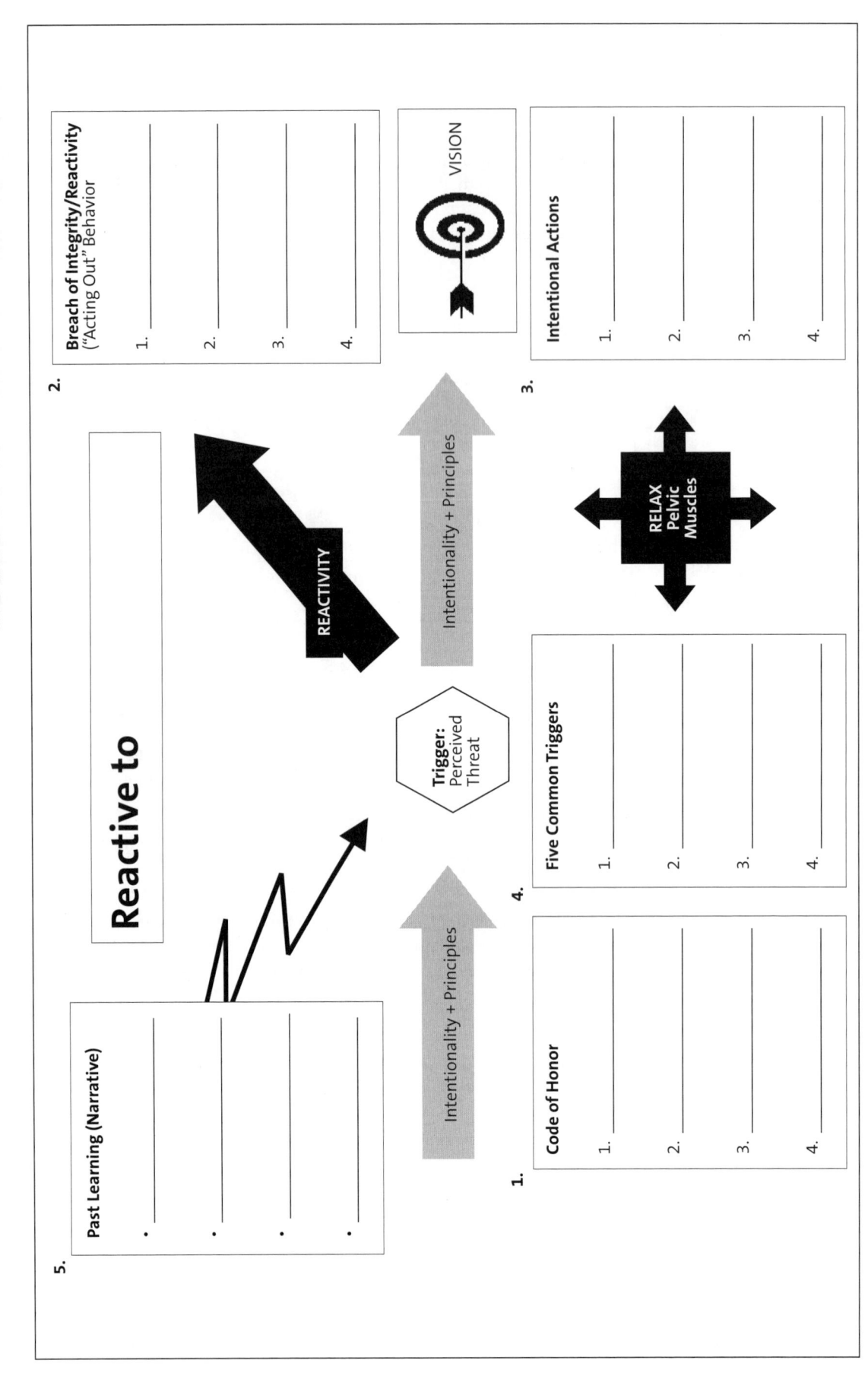

2. Breach of Integrity/Reactivity ("Acting Out" Behavior)
1. _____
2. _____
3. _____
4. _____

VISION

3. Intentional Actions
1. _____
2. _____
3. _____
4. _____

Reactive to _____

REACTIVITY

Intentionality + Principles

Trigger: Perceived Threat

RELAX Pelvic Muscles

4. Five Common Triggers
1. _____
2. _____
3. _____
4. _____

Intentionality + Principles

1. Code of Honor
1. _____
2. _____
3. _____
4. _____

5. Past Learning (Narrative)
- _____
- _____
- _____
- _____

Appendix 4
Training Opportunities

For up-to-date information on training opportunities and to arrange for training at your location, contact:

Dr. Anna B. Baranowsky
Executive Director
Traumatology Institute (Canada) Training & Development, Inc.
45 Sheppard Ave E., Suite 419
Toronto, Ontario Canada M2N 5W9
Tel. 416-229-1477 ext. 235
Fax. 416-229-9882
info@psychink.com
http://www.psychink.com

Online training is now available at http://www.ticlearn.com.
Visit http://www.traumaline1.com for a listing of trauma trained therapists, responders, trainers, and resources.

J. Eric Gentry
Compassion Unlimited
3205 Southgate Circle,
Sarasota, FL 34239
Tel. 941-720-0143
info@compassionunlimited.com
http://www.compassionunlimited.com

Online training is now available at http://www.traumaprofessional.net.

For organizations or teaching institutions that would like more information about the full Traumatology Institute Training Curriculum (TITC), please contact the Traumatology Institute (Canada). The TITC is a comprehensive set of training programs for developing specialization in the area of posttrauma response and recovery. The TITC is internationally recognized by the American Academy of Experts in Traumatic Stress and the Academy of Traumatology – Commission on Certification and Accreditation.

We would be happy to discuss options to becoming a fully recognized provider of the Traumatology Institute Training Curriculum.

The full TITC is available for qualifying organizations or institutions who would like to establish recognized site licenses through the Traumatology Institute.